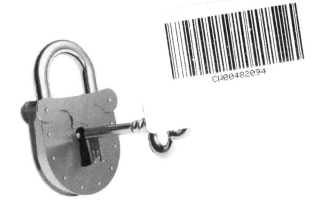

UNLOCK YOUR MAXIMUM
WEIGHT LOSS POTENTIAL

YOU ARE NEVER OVERWEIGHT FOR THE REASON YOU THINK YOU ARE!

FIND OUT HOW TO IDENTIFY THE REAL REASONS YOU CAN'T LOSE WEIGHT AND BE SLIM FOR LIFE!

Ann Parker

By the same author

Unlock Your Pet's Maximum Potential

How to communicate with, train and heal your pet: a complete guide

A must for all animal lovers and those with pets

Unlock Your Maximum Potential

A complete guide to attracting the life you have always desired

A must for children and adults alike who want to attract success and abundance

Disclaimer

The healing services and information offered in this book are for information purposes only and are not intended as a substitute for visiting the vet or doctor. Ann is not a vet and is not a licensed practitioner. Ann's healing work with people and animals should be understood as a positive and complementary therapy to professional medical care. Ann always recommends that people continue to work with and/or consult with their vets and doctors. Ann recommends that you continue to follow medical treatment as prescribed by your chosen healthcare professional. Ultimately you are responsible for your own and your pet's medical treatment and care, you are the one that makes the decision and Ann accepts no liability.

For entertainment purposes only.

Contact Ann Parker at
ann@annparker.co.uk
www.annparker.co.uk

Acknowledgements

I would like to send my love and thanks to everybody that has supported me over the last eighteen years but particularly to the following people who have all had their roles to play in my healing and recovery:

My Husband
To my husband Don who termed the phrase 'Oogie Googie' for everything spiritual, has always let me pursue my interests and never once complained!

My 'Oogie Googie' Friends
These are the friends who understood exactly what I was going through on this path which started as weight loss and ended up as so much more:
Valerie Rose, Angela Orban
Amanda Brooks and Sue Harris

To my best friend Margaret Kemp for her hours of proof reading and pointing out how bad my grammar is!

To my Mother, my beloved Jack Russell, Oliver, my beautiful Norwich Terriers Milie and Stanley, and Lulu, Hardy, Polly and Monty my Norfolk Terriers
You have been my biggest teachers and I thank you so much for everything I have learnt from you

To all my guides
I thank with all my heart my guides, angels and goddesses that have been wonderful in selecting me from the millions of people they could have chosen!

Special thanks to my main American Indian guide White Arrow, and to my animal spirit guides, one of which is a huge, silver backed gorilla called Papa Doc, who is my rock and Trixi, a faun, who is my lightness.

Section 1

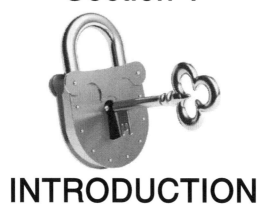

INTRODUCTION

Chapter 1:
WHY I HAVE WRITTEN THIS BOOK

Everything that is written in this book is gleaned from my own personal experience over the last 60 years. I am not a writer and I am certainly not a doctor either. The book is written in my own 'chatty' style and in layman's terms that, I hope, gets enough information over without being too technical (or boring) as there are masses of subjects to cover.

If you want to know more about any subject, there is a wealth of information now, both in books and on the internet, and I give a suggested reading and internet site list at the end of this book.

This book covers a myriad subjects from health to past lives; from hormones to karma; from hypnosis and meridian therapies to life coaching. Everything I have experienced in past years, including all techniques and therapies that I have found to work either for me, clients or close friends who had a weight problem, are in this book.

I have so much experience that I just want to be able to pass it on to people who are suffering in the same way that I suffered, by not being able to lose or keep the weight off, despite what I did. This is the ultimate in weight loss and if I can make one person feel better about themselves then I have done my job! The good news is that the words in this book have been filled with healing energy so you will now gain insights into why you can't lose weight and the blocks and resistance will disappear as by magic.

I feel very strongly about this now because people are so judgemental and rude to people who have a weight problem and this is why it is important for you not to judge other people or yourself. The worst comment I think is when somebody says "why Ann, you are truly beautiful on the inside!" What they mean is that you are ugly and fat on the outside! I feel this is patronising but it is important that you don't take offence with what people say to you and it is a good idea to have a couple of retorts that you can snap back. My favourite is "you are very rude and I would never be personal about you – and I could be!"

The biggest turning point in my life came when I asked myself if I wanted to lose weight and got the biggest shock when the answer came back as a definite "no". I was absolutely gobsmacked and couldn't believe it but it did explain why I was heavier than ever, as every time I tried something new the "no" would automatically kick into action because it wanted me to stop. So I believe you need to look at all aspects of your life including emotional, mental, physical and spiritual and this way you will 'lighten up' your entire life.

When some people lose weight and then stop dieting they seem to put it all back and more. The doctors come up with lots of explanations for this including starvation mode, going back to the same old way of eating, or greed. Having lost a considerable amount of weight, I would disagree with them all. You don't spend months dieting and exercising only to put everything back on again. You would perhaps put on a stone or two and then you would do something to take it off immediately. Remember, you would have all your new, smaller clothes and feel good wearing them, so you wouldn't want to go back into your old baggy ones, would you?

I believe that it is your subconscious that springs into action, almost as if you are asleep and wake up when all the weight has gone back on again. I see it time and time again and I have experienced it many times. So you need to find out why your subconscious doesn't want you to lose weight and how it is manipulating your body and your mind to stop losing weight or putting it back on immediately. This process is what the book explains in many different ways - how you can lose and keep the weight off for life.

As I am editing this section our annual TV programme, I am a celebrity get me out of here, is on. The campmates have been in for over 10 days now and showing off their slimmer frames. There is a lovely, larger lady called Anne Hegerty (one of the clever Chasers) who hasn't lost any. Now she, in theory, should have lost more than anybody else. This is a perfect example of the subconscious not wanting to be slim.

After all, the Hollywood lovelies cut their calories and don't put the weight back on. I also know lots of slim and medium size people who overeat, eat emotionally and don't exercise. If you look in pizza and burger restaurants, not everybody is overweight and they are eating the same thing - and I doubt that they are going home to have a sprouted salad in the evening!

The new way of tackling this current wave of obesity is surgery and this surgery is very invasive. A multimillion pound industry has now been set up for the surgery and it is being sold at every opportunity.

The problem is that the surgery dramatically cuts the calories the body can take in and can cause malnutrition, so it does mean that you could still eat chocolate at every meal but you wouldn't be healthy! What the doctors fail to see is that if somebody overeats there is a reason for it – it may be that there is no love in their life, or no sweetness or that they hate themselves. If these issues are not addressed, the weight loss surgery will not be successful. I have seen people become anorexic because they haven't healed their emotional problems or, even worse, have died. A lot of my weight was to do with protection, so if I suddenly removed this my subconscious was sent into panic and would devise another way to protect itself – in my case this was with excess water.

It is the same with the food industry, but despite billions of pounds and countless 'low calorie' products, people are still getting heavier.

You hear that scientists are trying to find a pill so people can eat what they want and not put on weight – and of course this will make the companies a fortune! But so far weight loss pills have not been successful and have many side effects. Also if you eat what you want you may still die as, although you may be slim, inside you may be fat and unhealthy.

Why are portions so big nowadays and why do people have to eat them?! Having said that it is also our beliefs that make us put on weight. If you think something you eat will put on weight it will! When I go out for dinner and see people noshing their way through three fattening courses and alcohol I know that most of them are not thinking that they are going to put on weight. However, I thought that with every mouthful I ate. Also if you keep focussing on saying "I am fat" you will be, as your subconscious will think that you want to and will oblige!

In no way is this book intended as a medical manual and if you have any type of health problem you must consult a qualified doctor or health care practitioner. However, what I am trying to succeed in doing is for you to take responsibility for your own problems, either health and/or weight, and be able to choose intuitively which avenue to follow, be it homeopathy, herbs or something else.

Don't rely on doctors and challenge everything they say to you as they don't understand how the metabolism works and everybody is different - do your own research and stick to your guns! I wish somebody could have done that for me twenty years ago and I would have saved myself in excess of £250,000 – yes, £250,000! That is what it has cost me to visit a multitude of therapists, buy the pills and remedies and, in some cases, train in that particular therapy if I thought that it should become part of my tool box.

What you will end up with, like me, is a great big Mary Poppin's type bag which holds all your learned therapies and techniques. Every day you dip into your bag and pick out the therapy or the technique that is right for you on that day. I don't believe that one type of treatment can heal you; instead I believe that you have to address every aspect of your being, emotionally, spiritually and health wise. Then your own self-healing mechanism will kick into place and you will become that healthy, slim and attractive person that you deserve to be.

I wish you all the luck in the world on your journey and remember you are never alone – you always have me! If you have an amazing weight loss story to tell, why not email me and let me know.

What's next?

I have put my heart and soul into researching all the subjects in this book and it has taken me over seventeen years and an incredible amount of money. As my mother would have said, I am now the most qualified unemployed person in the world! So am I going to put my feet up and retire? I think not!

Metabolism

The one question that I cannot get answered to my satisfaction is what does control the metabolism? People say it's the thyroid or it's carbon dioxide or it's insulin or it's how you breathe. My gut instinct is that all of these things are important but not the definitive answer – I have also felt that there is something missing and this has shown up in my research time and time again. My holy grail is what exactly controls the metabolism and how can I ensure that everybody's metabolism works at 100% and I won't be satisfied until I achieve this. So watch out for my next book!

Other subjects in the next book

- I also want to research the cosmetic surgery available for weight problems, including non-invasive techniques that are easier on the body.
- I want to perfect beliefs, so that your skin snaps back immediately you lose the weight, as the hanging skin that is left after weight loss is becoming a real problem
- I want to show you how to look good at any size by using the correct colours, clothes, hair styles and makeup – this is all so important to you looking and feeling good about yourself.

My wish for you

May you find serenity and tranquility in a world you may not always understand

May the pain you have known and the conflict you have experienced give you the strength to walk through life facing each new situation with courage and optimism

Always know that there are those whose love and understanding will always be here, even when you feel most alone

May you discover enough goodness in others to believe in a world of peace

May a kind word, a reassuring touch, a warm smile be yours every day of your life, and may you give these gifts as well as receive them

Remember the sunshine when the storm seems unending

Teach love to those who know hate, and let that love embrace you as you go into the world

May the teachings of those you admire become part of you, so that you may call upon them. Remember, those whose lives you have touched and who have touched yours are always a part of you, even if the encounters were less than you would have wished. It is the content of the encounter that is more important than its form

May you not become too concerned with material matters, but instead place immeasurable value on the goodness in your heart

Find time in each day to see beauty and love in the world around you

Realize that each person has limitless abilities, but each of us is different in our own way. What you may feel you lack in one regard may be more than compensated for in another

What you feel you lack in the present may become one of your strengths in the future. May you see your future as one filled with promise and possibility

Learn to view everything as a worthwhile experience

May you find enough inner strength to determine your own worth by yourself, and not be dependent on another's judgments of your accomplishments

May you always feel loved.

Author Unknown

Chapter 2:
MY LIFELONG STRUGGLE WITH MY WEIGHT

This is a story of my lifelong struggle with my weight which took a great deal of tenacity and money over sixty years to resolve. However, it was the best training course that I could have ever been on because as far as weight problems are concerned, I have experienced every aspect that you could possibly imagine. This is why I want to pass on my experience to other people. I come with empathy, love and understanding and will never say what I had been told over so many years "you eat too much" as I believe that weight and water retention issues are far deeper than food and these issues have to be resolved before any weight is lost and that loss is maintained.

Many times during these sixty years I have felt like giving up and sometimes committing suicide because I felt so totally out of control and it didn't matter what I did as nothing made any difference. There was very little support but luckily in later years I had some marvellous mentors who virtually saved my life. Most of my friends didn't even know what I was really going through and most would have thought me mad if I had told them what I am going to tell you.

Did you know that one in five people (especially women) suffer with underactive thyroid problems and most of those go undetected? Especially in the UK the only treatment offered is thyroxin and that is normally given if you put on weight suddenly. If you are already overweight there is very little support – the doctors blame food intake.

My Story

When I was born I weighed 12lbs (5 kg) and my mother gasped "that fat baby is nothing to do with me!" That started her obsession with my weight which, in turn, started my obsession. I was born in Karachi, Pakistan in a temperature of 110ºF with the cord around my neck and I nearly died – I must have known how difficult life was going to be! The doctor who delivered me had offered to abort me seven months earlier but my father wouldn't hear of it. So here was I, a fat baby, born to a mother who didn't want me as she had a wonderful social life with which I would interfere. She also had a weight problem which she didn't have before and blamed me for that as well! Incidentally I was born at a Mahjong party, as nothing as minor as childbirth would have put my mother off socializing!

When I was six months old I had whooping cough and dysentery which meant I couldn't eat for a considerable time but I didn't lose any weight. When my teeth came through, they came through crooked and bruised so once again there was a long period when I couldn't eat but once again I didn't lose weight. Now are you beginning to see the pattern?

But looking at pictures of myself as a small child I was plump, not fat. In a photo aged three I looked pretty, cute and gorgeous. However, I was aware of my weight as early as I can remember and knew my mother had a real thing about it. She talked about it all the time. I think this was also due to the fact that my mother had been slim until she had had me and therefore in some way blamed me for her extra weight as well.

I would say that I was on a diet from the moment I started to eat solid food. I was brought up on very small meals of light foods. I remember poached egg on toast and fish finger salad. Even as a child I knew that a fish finger contained only fifty calories. In those days most people would cover their vegetables in butter: we only ate them once a week on a Sunday but, of course, with no added butter. We ate salad most days without dressing but with a small spoonful of salad cream: salad cream is something with which I have an obsession and carry a jar in my handbag! I had skimmed milk and saccharine in hot drinks. I did not eat breakfast, ate no snacks between meals, had fruit for lunch and a very small meal in the evening. I wasn't even allowed pocket money in case I bought sweets and I have never had an Easter egg in my life!

My mother watched every mouthful I ate and would constantly comment on it. She first consulted a doctor about my weight when I was four and she was told that I was fine and I would slim down. I was also brought up to believe that illness was a weakness and you never complained or talked about how you felt so I just kept going, even when I felt really bad. I was also brought up that doctors are god and that you never disagree or argue with them.

So as you can see from an early age I was led to believe that eating wasn't good and that protein was the enemy because it was deemed as fattening. From around the age of six I was on 800-1000 calories per day with at least an hour's exercising, limiting my calorie intake the whole time under the watchful eye of my mother. My mother bought me books on exercising and insisted that I had to do these exercises every night and would hold the book and tell me what to do.

My sister, however, was not subject to the same regime and we were often compared. "It's such a shame about Ann because Susan is so slim and attractive" did nothing for my self-esteem!

However, leading up to an early puberty at 10½, I really did start to put on weight which gave my mother permission to exercise more control over me and my calorie intake was lowered even further. But much to my mother's horror, whatever I did didn't result in any weight loss. I suppose that this was the first time that I felt the 'out of control' feeling that was to haunt me later in my life. It also gave my mother the excuse to belittle me, so my self-confidence and esteem fell even further. I was such a disappointment to her and she told me that frequently.

My father was in the Royal Air Force so in the first fifteen years of my life we lived in over twenty different houses in the UK and different countries. I attended four different grammar schools (twelve schools in all) but I remember the embarrassment of always being the new girl and, to make it worse, often had to have my uniforms specially made for me when the available sizes didn't fit. Also my mother made all my other clothes which again increased the control she had over me and gave her the opportunity to ridicule me even more.

Although being the 'fat' new girl at so many schools, luckily I was never the subject of bullying and because I have a bubbly personality I always made friends easily, except boys were never interested in me. It was fortunate that there was only one school I didn't like and I was so unhappy there that I threw myself down the stairs hoping to get a few days off. However, I didn't hurt myself and was sent back immediately!

This change of schools affected my exam results quite dramatically as the curriculum is not the same in different counties, let alone countries, which means that I did the first year of German four times but missed out huge chunks of other subjects that I needed. My grammar and spelling are not brilliant (as you will find out!) but this is down to the constant change in teaching. Unfortunately this added further to my mother's disappointment in me, which she voiced all the time. Now I was fat, ugly AND stupid so my self- confidence and esteem went down even further.

As my parents were older than most parents of their generation and had a busy social life, I also mixed with a lot of adults, rather than playing with children of my own age. As a child I was either sitting quietly at a coffee morning or handing out drinks at a party. Because of this I have always felt that I was 'born old' and never experienced much of a childhood. Even to this day I have no idea what children like or how to play.

Once some of the puppy fat had been eventually dieted away (by lowering my calorie intake even further), when I started work at seventeen I was a size 18 and started Weight Watchers, thinking that this would provide the solution. Not so. On a typical calorie-controlled weight loss program on which most people would lose weight, I would gain weight and my protestations were not heeded. "You are putting on weight because you are not following the program". Nothing could be further from the truth and this was to be repeated with Slimming World and the Cambridge Diet. In fact I got thrown out of Slimming World and Weight Watchers for putting on weight!

In hindsight I can see that a size 18 isn't particularly big for someone who is 5'8" tall with a broad build, enormous breasts and big thighs. So my figure was in proportion, with a flat stomach and a small waist, in other words I had a curvy figure. I was also told that I had a beautiful face but people would always finish it off with "but it is such a shame about the rest of you!"

Apart from the inability to lose weight I had a list of symptoms as long as your arm including severe constipation, acute tiredness, oedema, greasy skin and hair and three weeks PMS per month which resulted in horrendous water retention. Whenever I went to the doctor to ask for a thyroid test I was told that all symptoms related to me eating too much and because I had such a good head of hair it couldn't possibly be my thyroid. However, I come from a family who all have thick hair so that is genetic. The symptoms for a thyroid problem can be as many as 150 and you won't have them all – although I did seem to have most of them! As I was led to believe that doctors were always right, I didn't challenge this decision and continued to suffer. I remember begging a variety of doctors and even bursting into tears in one doctor's office as I was so desperate. So you can see why my opinion of doctors is very low and has remained that way for all of my life.

When I was 19, after a particularly strong battle of wits with my mother (which I lost!), I woke up one morning with Bell's palsy. This is where one side of your face drops and according to Louise Hay who is the author of *I can heal your life,* it relates to acute unspoken rage, which was just how I was feeling. It was frightening for a pretty, young girl to start dribbling. I was sent to an RAF hospital which most probably saved my face. They monitored me for a while and decided that as it wasn't getting any better they would operate. It's very unusual for an operation to be performed for Bell's palsy in those days. They scraped the nerve which I believe is a very dangerous procedure but luckily it was a success. Eighteen months later my face had returned to almost normal, to the eye anyway, although in a photograph my face looks crooked and when I am tired my left eye closes. This episode brought me back into the grip of my mother, my boyfriend ran a mile and I couldn't work for some time as not only did I have a crooked face but also no hair where it had been shaved off.

After my father died I went to Beauty College which I really enjoyed and that is why I am so interested in potions and treatments today – I always call myself an old beautician! However, when I left college I couldn't find a job in beauty so went back to secretarial. This was to be the making of me as I soon got involved with word processors and joined a word processing company doing training and support.

From there I progressed to computers and have had some fabulous jobs, travelling all over the world doing training, business analysis, product management and project management. I eventually went to work as a contractor, as the money was so good before Year 2K, which enabled me to pay for all this other training and treatments which I most probably wouldn't have been able to afford on a 'normal' salary. So strangely enough, although I have had this obsession with my weight, I have never had any doubts about my work ability.

When I was in my early twenties I went on the pill and this must have raised my hormone levels over the level that causes water retention. My PMS vanished and along with it my three weeks of hormonal water retention and sore boobs. This was like being set free. For the first time in my life I felt great and lost a considerable amount of weight. Unfortunately I didn't realise the consequences of this at the time and also that this had happened in the summer. This was my first experience of Seasonal Affective Disorder (SAD) and its affect on the body. I got down to a small size 16 and I had a ball with lots of boyfriends and it was at this time that I met my husband. However, I was still struggling to keep my weight down. By this time I was eating about 500 calories a day and I had developed an iron willpower.

When I moved in with Don I came off the pill and I started to cook a meal in the evening and I started to put on weight. I must stress that it was still a small meal for me and my other eating habits hadn't changed but all the hormonal water retention came back and the extra calories just tipped me over the edge. Once again I felt totally out of control because whatever I did made no difference what so ever.

When I was 31 my mother was diagnosed with advanced colon cancer – she died shortly after – and Don asked me to marry him. I visited a slimming clinic and went on slimming pills and diuretics (to lose water). I only lost 1½ stone in five months but it was enough to look absolutely gorgeous in a cream silk dress encrusted with pearls and for the first time in my life I loved looking at a picture of myself. I have now realised that I couldn't have been that fat in the first place but my belief was that I was – and everybody told me I was!

I stayed on slimming pills and diuretics for seven years and managed to reduce my size to a small 14. My face went very drawn and my collar bones stuck out dramatically but interestingly enough I still thought I was fat (because I believed I was fat). Even more surprising is that a lot of people still told me I was fat and acted accordingly, plus the scales confirmed that I was fat because according to the charts my weight was still obese. At this time I also went for liposculpture in a bid to slim down the top of my thighs but that operation went wrong. The surgeon took the fat from the wrong place and didn't finish the operation correctly so now I am lopsided. This was another desperate attempt to lose weight in an area that dieting and exercise wouldn't shift.

The weight loss was also due to the fact that I noticed that in the summer my PMS went completely and at that time I had a new job where I was driving round the country in the sunlight for many hours a day. I then noticed it came back in October which means that I couldn't lose any more weight until the following April. I then realised how much the sun has an effect on the hormones and started to research SAD in much more detail.

However my calorie intake got lower and lower to about 150 calories a day and the exercise time got higher and higher to about three hours per day. I was very clever about hiding my not eating and when I went out for a meal I would order a starter and then only eat half. One weekend I went away and ate nothing the entire weekend, whilst watching other people eat full English breakfasts and large dinners. I was worried because if I had eaten the same I would have put on at least 10lbs. I never drank alcohol then as it is a total waste of calories – and I still don't today because it is still a waste of calories!

Although I took laxatives because I was constipated, the laxatives increased and because I was becoming increasingly desperate, I started to make myself sick when I ate. Luckily for me I hate being sick more than anything in the world and this was very short lived. I want to make it clear that I did not binge in any way at all and I was just trying to get rid of the little food that I had eaten. So I don't know whether I can call myself bulimic as I didn't binge before I made myself sick and I can't call myself anorexic as although I starved, I was still well covered. I was also eating a pack of sugar free mints a day which are a laxative – I would gag to get them down but they were brilliant for getting rid of water through the bowel and keeping the weight down.

At 38 I came off the slimming pills because of the side effects and how dangerous they were and the weight started to go on, especially in the winter. I also gave up smoking and just to reiterate what an iron will I have, I only put on 1lb whilst giving up a 40 a day habit. Smoking does increase your metabolism and I found that this was the final nail in my coffin as far as weight loss was concerned, as my already poor metabolism was then dropped by another 200 calories a day.

So I decided to contact a private doctor and paid for a thyroid blood test. There are two main constituents of the thyroid called T3 and T4. In very simple terms the T4 is thyroxin and T3 is an enzyme that enables the thyroxin to be activated. The normal NHS test does not include any test for T3, but without sufficient T3, even if you show T4 in your blood stream, the thyroid will not function correctly. On my blood test results I had virtually no T3 and very little T4. At this time it was impossible to get T3 in England. The doctor talked about importing some for me from the United States which, at the time, was a complicated and expensive procedure, so I decided to go on Thyroxin. I was put on 400 mg per day, which is in fact a dangerous dose that could result in a stroke. Over a six month period it made absolutely no difference whatsoever, so at this point I gave it up as a bad job and decided to try alternative therapies.

From the age of 36 to 41 I trailed around at lot of alternate therapies, including homeopathy, herbs, acupuncture, iridology, meridian therapies and various forms of healing but none made any significant difference for any length of time. It was disheartening, even devastating (not to mention expensive!) to start each new regime with such hope only to end up with the message "our cures usually work, but not on you, so you must be doing something wrong, you must be overeating".

I then went on various courses, learnt how to dowse with a crystal pendulum, bought books and studied on the internet. I started treating myself with a homeopathic remedy and to my delight I started to lose 2lb a week. The water seemed to flow from me leaving my ankles and feet really slim. It was the summer time so I had no PMS so that added to my weight loss.

At 41 I decided to support my treatment by becoming a qualified Reiki healer (Reiki is a form of Japanese hands-on healing). This involves becoming attuned to the healing energy at three different times to become a Master. However, after every Reiki attunement my symptoms got worse which, for some unknown reason, I didn't connect at the time to Reiki. I started to put back on the weight very quickly and the homeopathic remedy I had taken so successfully before stopped working. I began to swell up at a horrendous rate and it appeared that every time I tried to do something that was 'good for me' my kidneys (especially my right kidney) would stop working and I would immediately swell up even more. This was extremely confusing and frightening and I felt more out of control and alone than ever.

Also, shock horror – my small appetite disappeared and I started wanting to eat more and then had the problem of cravings and not feeling full. Whereas before I never bothered about food, now I was working out how and when I could eat, and craving salty and fatty foods. This was totally alien to me and sometimes I wouldn't feel full. This I found quite strange as previously I would be full to bursting after five mouthfuls. So now I had the added conflict of craving food but not giving into the cravings and this was extremely hard.

I spent the next seventeen years and vast amounts of money in the quest for a cure through alternative therapies, including muscle testing and dowsing (both give answers to Yes/No questions), homeopathy which I still felt held the key, colour therapies, herbs, life coaching, hypnotherapy, essences - in fact, I think that I have tried almost every treatment available, and trained in many of them too.

From muscle testing and dowsing it became apparent that not only was my thyroid function dangerously low but so were my hypothalamus, pineal, pituitary and adrenal gland functions – in other words my entire endocrine system was malfunctioning. That is why Thyroxin didn't work for me and it doesn't work for many other people either. This in a funny way was a relief because least I knew that there was something seriously wrong with me and now I had more information to find a cure.

I then came upon the notion of self-sabotage and realised that what the Reiki was revealing was that some inner force was stopping me. This was another realisation and I had no idea at this time how powerful your subconscious is and how difficult it is to change its perception, especially to guilt, self-punishment and self-hatred. So what I had to find out then was why did my subconscious not want to get better as it appeared I was on a journey of self-destruction.

Several issues were identified which included severe mother problems, masses of fears, non-existent self-worth and self-esteem which formulated self-hatred and a major childhood problem related to sexual abuse. I worked hard on these issues using all the techniques I had trained in and the more I worked on them the worse I got. Some days my ankles would swell by as much as 4" and my fingers would swell so much that I would cry with the pain. My stomach would swell and be as hard as a board. My PMS got even worse, if that is possible, and I felt like a cloud was hanging over me. My hair and eyelashes were falling out. I was deficient in most vitamins and minerals and was anaemic. Looking back I really don't know how I dragged myself around and kept going – it was tenacity and an iron will.

Now I felt even more alone and out of control than I had ever done in my life, had put on six stone, mostly water and I also looked nine months pregnant which I found particularly hard as I had always had a flat stomach. The humiliation that I received at the hands of others about my weight was amazing. The main one was the reaction of men which I found quite amusing. When I was a gorgeous size 14 men were always chatting me up and now the same men would stare in the opposite direction and ignore me like I wasn't there (how fickle men are!).

Most therapists looked at me as if I was mad when I talked about my problems being down to self-sabotage because most people equate overweight with overeating. Therapists should know better!

During years of working on myself I realized that the sexual abuse I had suffered as a child had meant that I wanted to close down as a woman and didn't feel safe. This is one of the reasons for the weight gain but I also didn't want to wear makeup or nice clothes. I simply didn't think it was safe to be a woman. So the weight was protection. The protection was also bringing up other issues such a dates rapes – it was a comment by Helen Mirren that sparked that off. In my youth this happened many times when I was put in situations that made me vulnerable. Also the attention that I had got when I was slim and beautiful had made me feel very unsafe. So I basically closed down as a woman.

So during this time I have experienced every symptom and every emotion that people experience when they are overweight – and I have had plenty of humiliation as well. I have starved, over exercised, then tried to eat more to raise my metabolism. My self-esteem was low and I hated myself. Now I know that this can all be turned round – but don't expect a quick fix – if you are going to do this you need will determination and patience.

Because of this problem I have now trained in homeopathy, herbs, hypnotherapy, nutrition, EFT™, NLP, karma release, past life removal, emotional clearing, other forms of hands on healing, life coaching, counselling, animal communication (I also work with animals and their weight problems as well) and crystals. So you can see that I am highly qualified in helping you with your weight journey!!

I eventually released the self-sabotage, the excess water and most of the weight and now have a successful business. It was a tremendous 'weight' off my mind and for the first time in my life I felt at peace with myself. However, now I am not striving to be a size 12 but I am happy at the weight I have ended up as. I am a large 16 and no doubt will be trolled by people saying why aren't I slim? Now I am more concerned with being healthy and fit and nourishing my body. I can now accept and love myself whatever weight I am and after all the humiliation and embarrassment, I can now look at myself in the mirror without wincing or crying and if people don't like looking at me they don't have too!!!

Please let me help and guide you through your weight loss journey!

Chapter 3:
OTHER IMPORTANT REASONS WHY YOU CAN'T LOSE WEIGHT

I have written many chapters on most of the issues that can cause weight gain and why you can't lose weight or keep it off. I have created this section at the beginning of the book as, not only does it make fascinating reading, it also gives you an overview of general, rather than specific areas where you are unable to lose weight.

Most of the information here is very brief so I would recommend if you want to know more on any of these subjects, use the internet as a research tool, visit the recommended sites or read the recommended books. You need to take control of every aspect of your life, not just diet or exercise. If you want to confirm whether or not you have a problem with any of these issues, use your new techniques that you will learn whilst reading this book – self-muscle testing, dowsing or your intuition.

These are all proven reasons why you can't lose weight and I know this to be true because I and many clients have experienced most of them. Remember everybody is different so what doesn't work for some may work for others. People may be on their first diet or they may have dieted for years and that needs a different approach. All the techniques in this book will enable you to overcome all your problems, including the ones listed below. Let me know if your particular reason is not on this list and I will add it when I do a review in the future.

Lack of sunlight

We are being told to keep out of the sun and to protect ourselves with suntan lotion at all times. But the bottom line is that sunlight is absolutely necessary for health. Sunlight activates your pineal and other members of the endocrine system and it increases your serotonin levels, which in turn elevates your mood. It also activates your metabolism, which I can account for because, when I am in the sun, my hormonal water retention disappears and I also drop weight. It is also essential for the production of vitamin D.

The amount of vitamin D in the blood influences the functioning of a hormone called leptin, which tells the brain when the stomach is full. The obese produced a tenth less vitamin D than those of average weight.

I don't want to go into the ins and outs of skin cancer in this book and I am not recommending that you sit in the sun for hours. However, there is now some very interesting research on why skin cancer is on the rise and it is not necessarily anything to do with the sun (except getting burnt). The research shows that one of the reasons is the lack of oils in the body (take your fish oil tablets PLEASE!). The other reason is the chemicals in the suntan lotion which you apply to your skin and then heat up. I have had suntan lotion that has taken off my nail varnish and burnt a whole through paint into wood! If it does that to paint, what is it doing to your skin? For more information on this subject I would recommend that you check out my favourite website www.mercola.com and order some of Joe's recommended suntan cream.

Seasonal Affective Disorder (SAD) is caused by lack of sunlight and people who don't suffer from it don't know how lucky they are! From October to May you become depressed and want to hibernate. Even if you don't eat any more you are guaranteed to put on at least 7lb over the winter months, which is then difficult to get off again. There is a lot of help for SAD now but you need to recognise that you have it. I have suffered with SAD all my life and the difference in my mood, weight and water retention when I am in the sun is truly gobsmacking. I was the first of all the people I know with a light box.

So make sure that you get into the early morning/late afternoon sun as often as you can but make sure that you don't burn your skin. Remember, everything in moderation!

Illnesses can make you fat

Did you know that there are many illnesses that can make you fat? There are quite a few! I speak a lot in this book about an underactive endocrine system will pile weight on you but here are some of the others:
- Under active thyroid also called hypothyroidism
- Diabetes and Diabetes II
- Heart problems

- Syndrome X which is the precursor to Diabetes II and also called 'insulin resistance'
- Polycystic ovary syndrome (this is where you have cysts on your ovary)
- Menopause + any other hormonal changes
- Depression
- Stress
- SAD (which I talk in some length about in the previous section)
- Cushing's syndrome – this is where your adrenals push too much cortisol into your body
- Water retention – I have given this its own section below because it is a big subject

Water retention problems

These are much more common than you would think but are barely recognised by the medical profession and usually their response is to have a massage!

Lymphoedema is caused by your lymphatic system not working properly. Your legs and ankles will swell as well as the rest of you and you will look as if have elephantitis. It sounds funny but believe me it isn't - I have experienced it. Not being able to get a pair of shoes on because your feet swell up so much is no laughing matter.

Lipedema is another swelling problem but this time the legs look like bottles.

Oedema is quite common with thyroid problems and there are many other symptoms, including hormonal water retention. If you have a kidney or bladder problem it may manifest as water retention.

If you have any of these problems do cut down on salt and don't fall for the hype of drinking a lot of water, as it sinks to the lower extremities. Homeopathy is very good for these types of problems but please consult an expert doctor.

Other people don't want you to lose weight

Yes this can really affect your weight loss and you don't even know it! Obviously the other people are not doing it consciously but they have their reasons why they don't want you to be slim and attractive and because you are connected to them you will allow them to sabotage you.

Why do they not want you to lose weight?
- Your husband thinks you may run off or leave him
- Your friends would be jealous
- Your sister always wants to be better than you and wants you to feel inferior
- Your colleague doesn't want you to be promoted over them

In this book you will learn how to cut the cords between you and these people and release their negativity.

Negative programming when you are young

Were you always told to clear your plate and got into trouble if you didn't? Did you have to eat everything that you were given even if you weren't hungry? Where you told you had to clear your plate because of the starving children in Africa? Were you given food as a treat or to shut you up? Did your mother show love by over feeding you? Or did she give you food to shut you up?! This programming has carried on into adulthood with you and you automatically now have to finish everything on your plate and then look to food as a treat, love or comfort. Well you are an adult now and you can stop. Start by leaving a little bit on your plate until you feel OK with it and then leave some more. The techniques in this book will be able to reprogram you to healthy eating.

Your soul contract and other personalities

Before you are born you draw up a soul contract of all the lessons you want to learn in this life. This may sound odd to you but please bear with me until this subject is explained later in the book. This soul contract could be that you want to experience a health or weight problem. You are also made up of lots of personalities and parts that have got stuck somewhere from this life or previous lives. So you could have a 3 yr part that was sexually abused and it does not want to lose weight because it doesn't want it to happen again. You could have a 10 yr old part who heard the parents arguing over money and you think you still have lack. This is why it is such a complicated process to lose weight and keep it off. Each of these contracts, parts, personalities and other parts of you like your shadow side need to be healed and then the weight will drop off for good.

Portion control

Why is it that when you went to the States the size of a pizza would feed a family of four for a week and you were supposed to eat it for one meal on your own? This sort of portion has become expected everywhere and has now spread to this country and Europe. This alone has quadrupled the calories in one go! Cut down on your portion size and fill up with vegetables. If you don't like fruit and vegetables, change your beliefs so that you do. Why isn't a mango as tasty as a cream cake? I believe that it is far tastier and I know it is much better for me as well.

Why don't you share a mail course with a friend or take it home in a doggy bag? I don't eat meat but I love going to a carvery because of the vegetables but I bring the meat home as a treat for my dogs! In a three course meal you could be eating an excess of 5,000 calories and you don't need it any more if you are serious about losing and keeping the weight off!

The calorie recommendations are too high for what we do

The recommended calorie intake for men and women of over 2,000 calories was fine when we lived in cold houses and walked everywhere. We sit all day and we drive everywhere – gone has vigorous housework, walking to school or work and is replaced by labour saving devices, cars, lifts and computer games. Unless you are eighteen, very active and with a good metabolism, the maximum should be nearer 1500 – even less if you are over forty. I believe these recommendations are being revised down but I haven't seen the results yet.

I recently saw a program with Jo Frost (super nanny) on what children should eat. I think that she is amazing and I am interested in everything she does. She sat the children round a table and asked the parents to give them lunch. There was a small pizza and every parent gave their child the whole pizza. A nutritionist then came on and said that the actual portion size was a quarter of the pizza! This is what they required for their development and growth, so it is not surprising that are children are starting off overweight.

There is also a lot of inaccurate information about what is good for you or what is low calorie – this is something I speak a lot about in this book. Sushi that you buy from supermarkets is not low calorie and it contains hardly any fish!! It is full of sticky rice which is quite calorific – so before you buy a pack for lunch please consult the calories! A big supermarket chain has recently decided to display their calories for their restaurant food – what a great idea. Would you believe that two different bowls of soup, chicken or minestrone, are nearly 500 calories!! This is because they use fatty stock and fry the vegetables. This doesn't even include the roll to go with it!! This is why I say you have to be careful what you eat and knowledge is power!

Every 10 years you should aim to cut your calories intake by 10%, because as you age, your body is less efficient and you are not so active.

We are not so active

Women are cutting down on housework and have labour saving devices. Children used to cycle or walk to school. Now we sit in a car, an arm chair or at a desk and very rarely move any part of our bodies! Some adults and children are playing computer games until 4am. School activities and sports have been cut down. As families, you can get out and about, walking or getting involved in sports, getting a lot more exercise which is fun to do together. I always try and make my housework and gardening a workout! You and your family need to get moving for your ongoing health.

Lack of willpower – No more excuses!

Years ago we always talked about having willpower! I gave up a 40 a day cigarette habit and I put on only 1lb, due to my iron willpower. What I notice these days is that people don't seem to have willpower anymore. They either want somebody to do everything for them or they give up at the first hurdle. I hear comments like "It is too hard and I can't do it", "I couldn't say no to the piece of cake", "I am on holiday so why shouldn't I eat what I want?" What about this statement – **'The taste of being slim is better than anything you can eat'**.

Lack of willpower also applies to exercise – I have heard all the excuses. My view is that if you have time to watch television you have time to do exercise. You could cycle or use arm weights while watching your favourite soap?! You just need to make it fun so you continue to do it. More about this is in the chapter on exercise.

If you lack willpower use EFT™ or self-hypnosis to give you a boost so, you can say 'no' and feel very happy about it. I know a lot of people who started smoking again, saying they were stressed but this is just an excuse. Smoking actually doesn't help stress and makes you more stressed – if somebody I loved died tomorrow, having a cigarette would not make me feel better. With dieting you need to take one day at a time because this is not a diet, it is a healthy eating plan for life. If your subconscious does not want you to lose weight it will absolutely kibosh your willpower. So you need to identity what is going on and heal it with something like EFT™.

If you have no willpower it could be your kidney energy that is low. In Chinese acupuncture the kidneys are responsible for willpower so you need to find an acupuncturist that will help raise the energy level which in turn will raise your willpower - **no excuses now**!

Not asking our body what it wants

In this book I discuss many times that we need to be really in tune with our body and our intuition. We "think" we know what is best for us but we never consult our body or our body elemental (more about that later in the book). So you go on a juice diet because you think you need to but does your body want to? Or you eat donuts – but does your body want that fat and sugar? You go to a boot camp and suddenly do 12 hours of exercise a day which totally knackers your body and you are so still you can't walk. Does this sound familiar? Your body knows what it needs so before you do anything – and I mean anything – you must tune in and ask your body. So before I eat or drink anything, before I exercise or before I take a supplement I ask is this good for me and then I act accordingly. I got very excited about Kefir (probiotic yoghurt) and I started to take it every day without asking my body because I assumed it was good for me and I needed it every day. So guess what after a week I was crippled with pain and I suddenly remembered that I hadn't asked my body how often I should take it! I had asked if my body needed it and it said YES so I assumed it meant every day. So I asked my body how often it wanted me to take kefir and it said twice a week. This is especially important when you are taking supplements and remedies because you won't need them every day.

A friend of mine went for a body treatment for her ME and the doctor recommended that she did particular exercises twice a day. I said this was too much and she should ask her body, but she believed she needed this frequency and she carried on. Within three days she couldn't move and was in tremendous pain because her body could only cope with the after effects twice a week. So it doesn't matter what you are told you must always check with your body!

Doing what you love

Whenever you do something you don't like your body will set up a stress response which could cause you to put on weight or become ill. So if you are dieting but eating what you don't like you could still put on weight!; if you are jogging to get fit but hate jogging you could be putting on weight!; if you don't like your job or you are doing something you don't like you could be making yourself ill.

So if you are dieting or trying to get fit it is essential that you do what you like. So if you don't like the gym find an exercise tape you love or do your gardening or housework with more vigour! If you don't like salad be creative with vegetables and include them in recipes so that you can't see them!! If you hate your job you really need to look at what you can do to change it or make it more pleasurable. You can always use EFT to change your beliefs so you like exercise and salad!

BMI and weight charts

When I was so slim that people started to worry about me, I was starving myself because, according to the weight charts that the doctors have, I was still obese – and the doctors were still telling me I was! So don't take too much notice because people are different body types, different bone densities and have different frames.

BMI calculations have now been shown to be totally useless and inaccurate for most people. This is why 'normal' children are now being sent letters to say they are obese.

So don't go by what somebody tells you or what the charts say as this can make you depressed or you may give up. Go by how you feel, how fit you are and how your clothes feel.

I used to get upset if I had to buy a dress size that I deemed to be too big. Then I discovered that I was a different dress size in various different shops. In the younger shops I would sometimes have to buy a size 18 and in M&S it would be a size 12! Now I take no notice of what size the outfit is, only how I feel!

New food types

Fizzy drinks – these are lethal for you and you should limit them dramatically, especially if you have children. They are either full of sugar and fattening or full of sweeteners and dangers. They are responsible for a lot of the weight problems and add a lot of extra water to the body.

Because they cause weight problems, avoid eating biscuits and crisps, plus anything else that contains transfats, colours or additives. Cut down sugar in your diet as well – read all the labels including baked beans and cereals – you will be amazed as to the sugar!

Prepackaged food, junk food and takeways – people say they haven't got time to cook so they are picking up this type of food. These are full of transfats and preservatives which cause weight gain and then you normally cook them in a microwave which then destroys any goodness at all.

There is now a multimillion industry around smoothies and juices – these are full of sugar and not only raise your insulin but ruin your teeth!! Don't follow what the industry tells you do your research and work out what is better for you!

Try to go back to cooking things from scratch – you know, it really doesn't take long to make a salad or cook a couple of vegetables and grill a piece of chicken.

Malnutrition, yo-yo and exhausted dieting

With food being the way it is you can actually eat a lot but still be malnourished. As you have learnt from this book, if you don't have the correct vitamins and minerals you will not be healthy or lose weight.

In the UK, rickets are making a comeback because children are fed on nuggets and crisps. Behavioural problems are rife because the brains are not being fed with the oils they need. Obesity is on the rise because of the food that is being eaten. This is really a wake-up call.

So if you are a yo-yo or exhausted dieter, you are also totally deficient in the oils, vitamins and minerals you need. If this is you, you won't lose weight! Start eating nutritionally and supplement where appropriate.

Fat virus

Why does everybody laugh when you talk about this – I suppose it does sound unlikely but why not? We have major viruses now that attack all parts of the body and weight management is such a complicated issue why couldn't a virus interfere with it?

Dr Nikhil Dhurandhar thinks that this virus does exist and has some intriguing research findings to back him up and is now working at Pennington Biomedical Research Center in the States.

Dr Dhurandhar's story starts in Bombay in the 1980s with a mysterious epidemic that wiped out hundreds of thousands of chickens. The birds were found to be infected with an adenovirus called SMAM-1. Adenoviruses are very common.

What was intriguing about the Indian chickens with SMAM-1 was not so much that they were probably killed by an adenovirus infection, but that they died plump, with a large, pale liver and large kidneys. They weren't thin and emaciated as you might expect an animal with a virus to be. Dr Dhurandhar deliberately infected some more chickens with the same virus and, sure enough, these birds also put on weight.

As he wasn't allowed to import any sick chickens into the USA, Dr Dhurandhar borrowed a human adenovirus, called Ad-36, from the US collection and set to work infecting first chickens and then rhesus monkeys and marmosets. Like the chickens, infected animals started to put on weight. Six months after they were infected, three male marmosets put on three times as much weight and doubled their body fat compared to three animals that were not infected. It was a very small study, but the results were still impressive.

I saw a television programme where a number of slim and overweight people were invited to a clinic in London and they were tested for the virus. The results were intriguing – none of the slim people had the virus but a third of the overweight people did. This shows that it isn't the main reason for obesity but could be one of the causes. There is no cure yet but I am sure that Dr Dhurandhar is working on one – I just wish he didn't have to do it on animals.

Interestingly enough, I am currently doing an edit on this section and discovered a piece on this subject in the Daily Mail, so it looks like the idea is now becoming more main stream – thank goodness for that!

Epstein Barr Virus

As I am editing this book, I have just discovered a fascinating man who calls himself 'The Medical Medium'. He is shown psychically immediately what is wrong with people and what to do to help them – and he is always 100% accurate. He has discovered that the Epstein Barr Virus is responsible for many things including ME, weight gain, inflammation and Lyme's Disease – and it could be responsible for many other illnesses. He says that the virus can hide so deeply in the body that doctors can't find it so can't diagnose the illness properly. There is more about this in the chapter on 'Organs'.

Other viruses and bacteria

An interesting New York Times feature examines the emerging research in infectobesity – the theory that microbes and viruses may be responsible for some causes of obesity. There seems to be a lot of research going ahead in this field. The latest piece I have read is that since the demise of helicobacter pylori (which caused stomach ulcers), levels of asthma, obesity and cancer of the oesophagus have been on the rise. It seems that the bug kept the appetite in check and the immune system strong. Take the bug away, the stomach acid rises unchecked and the appetite goes up and that can cause obesity. So the antibiotics should only be given to people who have no other choice. Interesting about the asthma, too.

It looks like some viruses may cause weight gain rather than the wasting away that is typically associated with this type of problem. I do talk about many viruses throughout this book so please don't disregard them!

These viruses and bacteria may be hidden and can be stored in many organs – mine were mainly in the thyroid and pituitary. I can help you identify these and help heal them.

Researchers in Shanghai studied mice that had been bred to be resistant to obesity. These mice remained slim despite being fed a rich diet and being kept from exercising. However, when some of these mice were injected with the human bacterium enterobacter, they quickly became obese.

Enterobacter was first linked with obesity after being found in high quantities in the gut of a morbidly obese human volunteer, said the report from Shanghai's Jiaotong University. The mice were injected with the bacterium for up to ten weeks as part of the experiment. The experiment shows that the bacterium 'may causatively contribute to the development of obesity in humans', according to the paper published in the International Society for Microbial Ecology.

So this is where it gets complicated because excellent article from the Daily Mail about gut bacteria doesn't mention enterobacter at all!!!! This is the article précised for you:

"We have lots of stomach bacteria and it is all very important in our health wellbeing and our weight. A company called Mapmygut will test your gut bacteria for you and then advise you on what diet to follow to improve the bacteria that is not in balance. Here are some of the bacteria that could be causing you problems with your weight. This could explain why you have trouble losing weight or gain it very easily – the lady in the article lost 3 lbs very quickly even though she had struggled before. Her low levels of certain bacteria meant that her body was ultra efficient in taking all calories from food and conserving them as fat.

- Ruminococcaceae – high levels of this bacteria is linked to obesity
- Rikenellaceae – high levels of this bacteria is associated with being overweight and linked to a high fat diet
- Akkermansia - should be 9-12% anti-inflammatory and improves blood sugar (the lady in the article was about 1%)
- Christensenellaceae - dubbed the skinny bacteria so if it is low trouble you will have trouble losing weight
- Bacteroidetes and firmicutes - good for extracting calories out of food which will add unwanted fat!

Same old diet advice really – avoid processed food and only drink a couple of times a week. Fasting is good as are fermented foods like Kefir and Apple Cider vinegar".

Brain cells

I recently came across this research which talks about brain cells causing weight gain – after all, everyone knows know slim people who eat cream cakes, chocolate and crisps!

Research article: *'An international study has discovered why some people who eat a high-fat diet remain slim, yet others pile on the weight. Researchers found in some people a high-fat diet causes the brain cells to become insulated from the body.*

Scientists say crucial brain circuits begin to form early in life so people may have a tendency towards obesity. This prevents vital signals, which tell the body to stop eating and to burn calories through exercise, from reaching the brain.

The team from Monash University, Australia, said the findings provide a critical link in addressing the obesity epidemic. Lead author Professor Michael Cowley, said: "These neuronal circuits regulate eating behaviours and energy expenditure and are a naturally occurring process in the brain. The circuits begin to form early in life so that people may have a tendency towards obesity even before they eat their first meal", he said.

Eating a high fat diet causes more 'insulation' in the nerve cells, and makes it even harder for the brain to help a person lose weight.

Professor Cowley said: "Obese people are not necessarily lacking willpower. Their brains do not know how full or how much fat they have stored, so the brain does not tell the body to stop refuelling. Subsequently, their body's ability to lose weight is significantly reduced."

Professor Cowley and his team collaborated with scientists from the Yale School of Medicine in the U.S, as well as teams from Cincinnati, New Jersey, Mexico and Spain. For a period of four months, the researchers monitored the eating and body composition of groups of mice and rats. They found that those with a neural predisposition to obesity gained thirty per cent more weight compared to six per cent of the group with obesity-resistant cells'.

Beliefs

You will find more information in the chapter on beliefs but it is important that you identify the beliefs that are making you fat and reverse them through affirmations and using EFT™ or self-hypnosis to make them positive.

Rebellion

Is there a rebel in you? When I used to smoke, the more people went on about me giving up the more I smoked! Is this the same for you with eating and getting fit? You may rebel because everybody is telling you what to do and you need to do it in your own time. However, let now be the right time as the longer you delay, the more damage you will have to undo.

A high set point

What is your set point? This is a genetically and biologically predetermined weight that your body tries to maintain. When you go below your body's natural set point, your metabolism will react and your body will start to sense it's in a state of semi-starvation and will try to use more effectively the few calories it receives. This is why some people lose weight and then either reach a plateau or regain it immediately.

When I went for some healing the guy said that my ideal weight was 12st 2lbs – this is the weight that I had tried to get below and couldn't. This healer came up with this weight so quickly that it must have been programmed into every cell of my body!

But don't worry because this can now be changed by me or you can use Emotional Freedom Technique, which is discussed in detail in this book. Decide what weight you would like to be and using then reset your set point to that weight – make sure that it is a sensible and healthy weight though.

Being Force Fed as a Child

I have been listening to Judy Satori's weight loss CD and she mentions resetting the appestat. I contacted Judy and this is what she says: *"When I talk about resetting the appestat I am talking about satiety levels and reducing craving for food. I believe that when a child is force fed it artificially pushes the natural satiety controls of the body up and that the sounds* (on Judy's weight loss CD) *to reset the appestat can assist in bringing this to normal.* Look at Judy's website, www.thesoundoflight.com - she has some excellent free MP3s to listen to. The CD certainly helped me and I could feel my breathing and my water retention changing as I went through the seven week cycle.

Also an intolerance to baby milk powder can set up a weight problem in later life.

Feeling small as a child

It has been found that if you are made to feel small, ignored, unimportant or inferior as a child and put down you can react later on in life by making yourself bigger to counteract this. This is your subconscious's way of making you be seen.

For various reasons my subconscious thought I was so much smaller than everybody else (inferior) that it over compensated with my weight and kept me large. It had totally got the wrong end of the stick and I needed to reverse the belief.

These problems are quite easily corrected by me or using Emotional Freedom Technique and positive affirmations.

Hiding away from the world

I know it sounds strange but your subconscious can actually make you bigger so that you can 'hide' and not 'be seen'! So this is another form of protection to keep you safe. Actually, as a large person, you and your views are ignored by most people and apart from commenting on your size, you become invisible – a bit like a woman over 50 even if she is slim!

You need to have counselling to identify why you want to hide away and heal the reasons.

Grief and coping with situations

Some people will lose weight when they are grieving or perhaps resort to alcohol or drugs – and some people put on weight. This is the same for emotional upsets or problems, people can react in very different ways. This is again the subconscious trying to protect you when you feel you can't control the situation.

One of the main reasons anorexics say they don't eat is because it is the only thing they can control in their lives. I must admit to this as when I lived my seven years on around 150 calories I felt great because I had total control over what I put, or didn't put in my mouth. This is just another way of coping and trying to control the situation.

Once again this can be reversed and healed.

Self-sabotage

I do cover this very widely as I am the queen of self-sabotage and have managed to sabotage my life quite dramatically over the years! There are many reasons for self-sabotage, including pushing people away, feelings of inadequacy and not good enough, being unlovable, not having to do something like moving forward or doing a job, or because you don't feel safe.

You need to stop self-sabotaging now and take control of your life!

Trauma and PTSD

Once again people react to trauma and PTSD differently but some people will react by over eating and/or putting on weight. There is a huge chapter on Stress that will give you all the information you need to have this healed as soon as possible.

Sleep apnoea

It has now been proven that this problem can cause you to be overweight and when you are overweight you suffer with sleep apnoea more! It is a vicious circle and you need to look at ways of curing it.

Not seeing yourself correctly

Recently, the London Mayor, Boris Johnston, looked at waxwork model of himself and exclaimed *"Am I as fat as that?"* People who have been slim very often don't see themselves as putting on weight until they see a particular picture of themselves. I know some people who are wearing clothes that are two sizes too small as they believe they are still that size! Likewise when I was slim I still saw myself as fat which is not good!

One of our greatest comediennes, Dawn French, said recently that she had 'fat blindness' and that this is starting to be recognised as a medical complaint: people could not see their weight.

Also if your friends or family are overweight you will be judging yourself by their standards and once again you will not be seeing the real you.

Dehydration

It is a well known fact that hunger can be mistaken for dehydration but did you know that mild dehydration could slow your metabolism down by 3%? That is quite an amount. Although you will know that I don't advocate the blanket 'eight glasses of water a day' message, it is important that you drink enough to keep you hydrated. This water should be filtered or bottled – if it is bottled it should be stored in glass and not plastic.

One glass of water shuts down midnight hunger pangs so if you are inclined to get those, sip a glass of water before you go to bed.

Use your diagnostic tools to ascertain how many glasses of water is right for you. Also remember, just because you drink water doesn't necessarily mean that you are hydrated. If you have a water retention problem (like me) the water could be going in between the cells and not nourishing the cells themselves. This can also cause hunger, as the cells are not being nourished with food.

Fidgeters are more likely to be thin

Scientists working in German and the US have found a fidget molecule and if you have it in your genes you are less likely to be fat. We all know fidgety people and chances are that they are slimmer – I also believe that this is linked to a high metabolism. So start to fidget!

Food as a reward

When we are children we are very often given food as treats or on days out – or sometimes to quieten us down and shut us up! So this means that in future we use food (or a bottle of wine!) as a reward for a hard day at work or as a comforter. When I am ill the first thing I want is a bowl of tomato soup because that is what my mother would have given me, so that is my comforter. Reward and treat yourself with something else that will do you good, such as book or a massage.

Lack of Sleep

You need a minimum of seven hours to keep your hormones regular otherwise too little sleep will interfere with your leptin and grehlin levels and you will feel hungry when you get up in the morning and will continue to binge all day. This could account for the rise in children obesity, as they seem to be up all night using their computers and playing games and starving the rest of the day. This could be because it also affects your blood sugar levels.

It looks like lack of sleep or irregular sleep may put your body into a state of high alert, increasing stress hormones and driving up blood pressure. In the chapter on stress I discuss at length the affect that stress has on weight gain.

Unexpressed anger and emotions

It would appear that if, when you were a child, you were not allowed to express anger towards someone, this repressed anger could be stored as fat (this is what happened to me). This is because the anger is not expelled from the body and the anger as fat then serves to protect you from that person in the future.

Also trapped emotions can be stored as fat and excess water. Grief manifests itself as water retention which is often expressed as unshed tears.

Eating too fast

Apparently those who wolf down dinner treble their risk of being overweight. It is suspected that the joint impact of eating too fast and eating until full overrides signals in the brain which would normally encourage a little more self control.

If you eat slowly then there is some feedback from the brain that tells you when you have had enough and this helps stop you eating before you are full.

However, I know lots of slim people who eat slowly but still eat everything that is on their plate – I also know slim people who eat very quickly! But do try to slow down, chew everything very carefully and know what you are eating – I know so many people that eat on the run and they can't remember what they have eaten!

Lack of satisfaction

Apparently if you get less satisfaction from eating you may eat more. Researchers from the University of Texas, Austin, took scans showing the flow of blood in the dorsal striatum part of the brain which deals with reward and pleasure. Then they tracked changes in the women's weight over the following year and the brains that responded the least to drinking a milkshake – and who got less pleasure from the treat – were most likely to gain weight. Make sure, therefore, that you eat things that you enjoy. And if you don't enjoy them change your beliefs so you do!

Being given the wrong information

There is so much inaccurate information out there I can't begin to tell you! The multimillion dollar businesses based on slimming are full of conflicting information. Smoothies and fruit juices are so fattening and will cause fat to be stuck around your middle. We have seen the research saying that sweeteners actually cause weight to be gained. Corn syrup is changing the metabolism for the worse. That is just the tip of the iceberg.

Some research says you have to eat your food raw – well my acupuncturist says no especially for me like me who have damp (yes I know it is very funny!!). Some say you have to graze or fast. What do you chose? This is why it is important to start to develop your intuition and become to really know you and what suits you the best. Challenge everything you hear as it may not be good for you and follow your heart.

Most countries have a food pyramid giving what % of general food types you should eat a day. Originally it contained mainly meat and vegetables and limited carbs and sugar. In the main people were very healthy. Then research showed that fats were bad for the heart so in the 80's it changed to limit protein and fat and upped the intake of sugars and carbs and this is when people started to put on weight. This research has now been shown to be inaccurate and that sugar and transfats are the real culprits so it is ok to eat eggs and meat – as long as it is in moderation. This shows how information that you think is correct can be so wrong for you so read the research and then make up your own mind.

pH Balance

Healthy people are slightly alkaline but unfortunately our diets are full of acidic foods such as meat, dairy, sugar and artificial sweeteners. pH stands for potential hydrogen and indicates when something is acid (below 7) or when something is alkaline (higher than 7). The pH of your blood must be between 7.3 and 7.4 and to protect the pH of your blood the body stores excess acid in fat cells. Therefore in an overweight person the body cannot afford to burn fat because it would release the stored acid into the system.

Eating plans like *The Hay Diet, Eat for your Type* and *Metabolic Typing* all use the principal of making the body more alkaline. This is a very important reason why some people cannot lose weight and although it is mentioned in the eating plan section, I would recommend that you use your diagnostic tools just to see how acid you are. As it is a very interesting subject, I would recommend that you do some more research and really become au fait with what makes you acid or alkaline. Remember that water is also essential to the body balance of pH. For the books and websites that I recommend for your information, go to the Recommended Reading section at the back of the book.

Some supplements can make you fat

Adding vitamin supplements, including folic acid and vitamin B12, to the diet of pregnant mice caused their off springs' weight to increase -- and the increase continued through generations. There has been further research that other vitamins may cause weight gain, such as oils and other B vitamins. This is why it is essential to check, with either dowsing or muscle testing, on everything that you take. You should also check how many to take a day and for how long.

Supplements can make you slim!

Sometimes not be able to lose weight (or being depressed) is simply that you are deficient in certain vitamins and minerals. Vitamin D has now been showed to have a dramatic effect on weight loss along with Omega 3 type oils. When you start you should be taking good supplements and then you can decrease as you get better.

Genetics

It is now being discovered that certain illness is genetic – so much so that women with breast cancer in their family are having their breasts removed.

Why then do people think that it is not true that build and weight can be genetic as well? You can have two siblings that are separated at birth and when they meet up in middle age they are the same build and size. This cannot be a coincidence and they cannot eat the same amount and type of food over the years that they have been apart.

Build and weight does run in families and you only have to look around to see this for yourself. Sometimes it can be caused by ancestral karma which brings you all together in this lifetime to release it.

You can all recognise certain races that have very small builds or are very tall – for example the Thais and Indians are very small boned whereas the Peruvians are shorter and have a larger frame. When I went to Polynesia I felt quite slim as the people there are generally of a large frame and quite chubby!

Just because it is genetic it doesn't mean though that you can't change it so no excuses!!

Obesity genes

There have been quite a few amazing discoveries recently and I am sure there will be more the years to come. Many people are trying to find a cure for obesity as it will make them very rich! However, a word of warning – obesity has many strings to its bow and one cure will not work for all, as has been found recently with the discovery of leptin. Leptin worked for some people but not all of those who are obese has trouble with their leptin levels.

Scientists have found a gene called gAD2 which speeds up the production of the chemicals that boost the appetite. This could cause you to want more to eat and will give into hunger more readily than other people.

Another gene called FTO has been discovered which is more likely to be found in people with Diabetes II. Research shows that those with the fat gene will be 70% higher risk of obesity that those with none and weigh 3kg (6.5lb) more if they have two copies of the gene, one copy being 30% risk of obesity. Research is now showing that this gene may give us a addiction to junk food, too.

Melanocortin-4 receptor gene (MC4R) can make suffers pile on the weight despite all their efforts not to overeat. This has just come to my attention through an article in the Daily Mail which shows twins – the boy is ultra slim and the girl is over twenty stone and it has been discovered that she has this gene. These sufferers also have more muscle and denser bones and looked big boned (sounds just like me!). Hopefully they will come up with a drug to counteract this gene.

The latest gene I have just read about on the BBC web page is the adipose gene. The University of Texas has manipulated this gene to alter the amount of fat tissue laid down by fruit flies, mice and worms – hopefully they can do this with humans. This gene looks like it could be a master switch and it decides whether it is going to accumulate or burn off fat.

Another faulty gene has been discovered - KSR2. Scientists at Cambridge University decided to investigate whether a gene called KSR2 was important for human obesity after researchers in the US showed that blocking the gene made mice profoundly overweight. The UK team looked at the genomes of more than 2000 severely obese people and spotted scores of mutations in the KSR2 gene. The gene is one of a group that governs how hormones such as insulin are used in the body and ensures that cells grow, divide and use energy properly. Lab tests found that mutations in the gene caused signals in cells to go awry and, in many cases, damaged their ability to process glucose and fatty acids, the body's energy sources.

The scientists found that people with KSR2 mutations had a greater appetite in childhood but a lower metabolic rate, so they consumed more calories and burned them slower than others. This discovery is very interesting as once again it shows that weight gain isn't all about being greedy.

Every month it seems that somebody is identifying another wildly important gene – I believe this is because companies want to be the first to market with the 'new cure' but I don't believe there is only one cure. New genes identified are Lpl, Lactb and Ppm11 – these all seem to promote fat gain, according to scientists in Seattle.

MGAT2 is an enzyme rather than a gene that has been identified. Scientists from the University of California have focused on an enzyme called MGAT2 which is found in the intestines in humans and mice. This enzyme determines whether the fat we eat is burnt off as energy or stored in the body. When tested on mice it appeared that the mice could eat a high fat diet while remaining slim and healthy.

Now scientists are trying to invent an exercise pill! US scientists have unveiled an experimental drug which fools the muscles into thinking they have worked long and hard boosting fitness and fat. Speaking as somebody who used to do three hours exercise a day and it didn't make any difference, I would like to see the results of this one!

Orexin is a hormone that prevents obesity in mice by activating brown fat and it is the brown fat that burns calories. This could explain why some people don't overeat but still retain the weight.

If there is a gene that I have missed out, perhaps you could email details to me and I can add it to my next review.

I can either activate genes or switch them off using my techniques so, if you think you are having problems in this area, please email me.

Stress can make you fat

Most people admit that when they're under stress healthy eating habits can be difficult to maintain. Whether eating to fill an emotional need or grabbing fast food simply because there's no time to prepare something healthy, a stressed-out lifestyle is rarely a healthy one. But weight gain when under stress may also be at least partly due to the body's system of hormonal checks and balances, which can actually promote weight gain when you're stressed out, according to some researchers.

When you are stressed adrenaline floods your system and unfortunately causes the cells to pump fatty acids into your bloodstream to give you the emergency stores of energy you need for the flight or fight action. So as you are not going to fight anyone, the fat stays in your blood stream and along comes the hormone cortisol to dump this fat around your stomach.

If you have a stress problem I would suggest that you buy my book, Unleash your full potential, which has an entire section on stress and is packed with great information so you never suffer again.

Medication

Research has shown that some medication can make you put on weight. For example, beta blockers, diabetes mediation, anti-depressants and allergy remedies can add a minimum of 20 lb to your weight. Women who have been on the contraceptive pill or HRT know how this can increase their weight and water retention. A cancer drug which is similar to progesterone is causing doctors concern by the weight gain it is causing.

There are other medications that can increase the appetite and make you gain weight so check with your doctor (or dowse) if you are unsure. Also, there are other medications that can slow down your metabolism. Steroids are renowned for putting on weight, encouraging you to hold onto water and then making it difficult to lose any weight. Anti-depressants can make you feel hungry all the time but you can still gain weight even if you keep your eating in check. If you think that your medication may be causing you to put on weight please check with your doctor and do some research on the net.

Scientists in Glasgow found that insulin for diabetes II can put on about 13 lb a year, while some drugs for epilepsy added more than 12lb, so it is not a fallacy – some medication can add weight and this can go on every year regardless. I have heard of young girls not taking their insulin because they don't want to put on weight and this is very dangerous.

Sleep eating

Yes, I know this seems like the biggest excuse of all times! Doctors are beginning to recognise a problem with sleep eating instead of sleepwalking (at least if you are sleepwalking you are burning off calories!). People can cram the most amazing amount of food into their mouths when they are asleep and don't realise it has happened unless somebody happens to see them – although they surely must spot the next morning that there wasn't the same amount of food in the fridge that there was the night before!

Obesity is catching!

Obesity could be catching. A US study found the risk of someone becoming obese was increased by 57% if their friend is obese. This trend follows with siblings (40%) and spouses (37%). The researchers at Harvard Medical School and the University of California suggest this is due to people's perception of an acceptable body size changing if surrounded by others of a larger shape.

Talking about obesity

Remember all the information regarding being careful about what you wish for and that your thoughts can become your actions? A psychologist from the University of Staffordshire believes that the constant avalanche of scary stories is making things much worse. All these stories make us more stressed about our weight which is one of the key triggers of comfort eating. Also, when things keep being discussed they become real – like the latest recession. We certainly 'talked ourselves' into that one! Remember to think positive thoughts and what affects other people does not have to have any effect on you.

Eating too much because you don't realise how much you are eating!

In the Daily Telegraph there was an interesting article, as follows:

'Slimmers began to eat healthier food when they were asked to take a picture of what they were eating, scientists found.

The pictures appear to have concentrated the dieters's mind at just the right time, before they were about to eat, the researchers who carried out the study believe.

Photographs were also more effective at encouraging volunteers to watch what they ate than traditional written food diaries.

To test if encouraging slimmers to photograph everything they eat might also encourage them to change their diet, scientists from the University of Wisconsin-Madison asked forty three people to record in pictures as well as in words what they ate for one week.

When the volunteers were later quizzed, the photo diary appeared more effective at encouraging them to change their eating habits to more healthy alternatives'.

The photographs also acted as a powerful reminder of any snacking binges, the researchers found.

"I had to think more carefully about what I was going to eat because I had to take a picture of it," was a typical response from volunteers, the scientists found.

Professor Lydia Zepeda and David Deal, the researchers who carried out the study reported in New Scientist magazine, found that written food diaries were often filled in hours after the meal and were not as powerful in creating an impression of how much food had been consumed.

"Nutritionists see diaries as recording tools. Now they should explore the role of photo diaries as intervention tools," Professor Zepeda said.

Frankie Phillips, a dietician with the British Dietetic Association, said that photographs could also help dieticians to identify if a patient is eating too large a portion size.

"Many patients tend to underestimate how much they are eating, especially when it comes to things like takeaway portions," she said.'

There is a fab health advert on at the moment where they show a family the amount of fat in a pizza – it is enough to put you off for life!

Use of Pollutants

Pollutants can interfere with the hormones that can lead to weight and water gain – more about this in the allergy section. Try to stop using all the creams, household products and anything else that is full of chemicals. Two things that really hit me and made me swell up were washing powder and air fresheners – air fresheners are particularly lethal and this can include scented candles as well. The other one is the coating that is put on carpets and settees and this is particularly bad for animals, too.

I had no idea how serious this problem was until I put air fresheners around the house to get rid of the doggy smell! Within 24 hours my ankles and stomach had swollen to record proportions and I had no idea why. It was when I had an allergy test and was told that air fresheners were like poison to most people and animals – and we all have them in our house.

Wash all fruit and vegetables to get rid of any pesticides. Air any dry cleaning to get rid of the fumes or don't have anything dry cleaned if you think you may have an intolerance. Make sure you are not using aluminium pots or too much tin foil. Try not to use food and drink in metal cans. Replace with paper bags the cling film that you use and buy water in glass bottles not plastic. Watch what you are putting on your body in the way of creams and lotions – try to go as organic as possible.

Also have your fillings replaced with white fillings because amalgam causes many illnesses and is now being recognised as a poison.

You can use certain products to get rid of all this poison from your body and Chelation therapy and hair analysis (see section on Other Therapies) is excellent if you have a serious problem.

Other Poisons that you use

Hand gel, shampoo, conditioner, body lotion, fluoride – you name it and it can poison you and affect the balance of your body. Then you can put on weight and may not be able to lose it. Hand gel is particularly lethal and can change the hormones and screw up the thyroid.

Please use body products and cleaning products that are as natural as possible.

How your body absorbs vitamins and minerals

I mention in the book how someone told me that I would find the 'missing link'. I was introduced to a hair analysis company (more info in the section on Other Therapies) and it showed the minerals and vitamins that were in my hair and then it worked out from various ratios how my thyroid, adrenals, metabolism worked and how I digested sugar and protein – it was truly amazing – and analysis of everybody that I have put through this process has been 100% correct.

They also give you masses of information of how to stop the poisoning – which is usually caused by lead, aluminium etc and very often comes from past lives which is why you don't think you are consuming these poisons now. Everybody I see has to have their hair analysed and then has to take the recommended supplements.

As the thyroid tests given by the medical profession are limited, people with a thyroid problem are sometimes told they don't have a thyroid problem when they have, so it's a shame that hair analysis is not recognised by the medical profession.

Smoking

Smoking can raise your metabolism by up to 300 calories a day – this does eventually sort itself out but not before you have put on weight! But give it up smoking now – the dangers of smoking are worse than excess weight.

Central heating and air conditioning

If it is too hot or too cold we burn calories to cool down or heat up. But if the temperature is just right the calories may be turned into body fat instead. We all have air conditioned cars and offices and beautifully heated houses so we are not using energy to warm us up or cool us down as we used to in the olden days. Make the relevant adjustments now and burn off more calories!

Living longer and other issues

We are living longer and tend to put on weight as we get older. Our organs slow down as we get older and are not so affective and this could cause weight gain. Just be aware that this is happening and start to make plans now so that you retain your youthful body function.

Snacking

A recent television program followed two young women in their daily lives and filmed what they snacked on. Believe it or not, they doubled their daily calories with their snacks and didn't realise it! They also thought they were snacking on healthy snacks which we know aren't healthy but full of sugar and fat! Snacking also becomes an addiction as the additives in snacks make the food so tasty you have to have it all the time.

When writing your journal, ensure that you include your snacks – or, preferably, stop snacking as it puts extra strain on your digestion and could cause inflammation. Mind you I do know slim people who snack a lot as well!

The new drinks

People are adding the new coffees into their daily routines and they appear to have no idea how many calories they contain – and believe me they are horrendous!! Some people have two or three a day!! I have also seen articles on low fat products where people recommend having a full fat latte – NO!! Always go for a skinny as you are not eating to make you full!!!!

Just for your interest this is the average calories/fat etc. of the new fancy drinks made with whole milk. All figures given here are based on averages in drinks made from whole milk (where relevant) from high street coffee chains.

Latte

What is it?   1-2 shots of espresso with steamed milk
Calories: Small, 200; large, 341
Fat: Small, 10.6g (6.6 saturated); large, 17.9g (11.2 saturated)
Verdict: Surprisingly unhealthy. A large latte contains almost one third of the daily recommended fat intake for women.

Add a vanilla shot and you add 380 calories and 14.5g of fat in each large cup. This is equivalent to ten rashers of bacon.

How to make it healthier: With skimmed milk – about 90 calories

Cappuccino

What is it?	A mix of steamed and foamed milk added to an espresso shot
Calories:	Small, 122; large, 207
Fat:	Small, 6.4g (4g saturated); large, 10.7g (6.7g saturated).
Verdict:	Better than latte but with 6.7g of artery clogging saturated fat in a large mug, it's hardly healthy.

How to make it healthier: With skimmed milk – about 100 calories

Hot Chocolate

What is it?	Chocolate drunk with whole milk, often topped with whipped cream
Calories:	Small, 357; large, 549
Fat:	Small, 18.7g (10.7g saturated); large, 27g (15.2g)
Verdict:	A large cup has the calories and fat content of three hot dogs, according to the Centre for Science in the Public Interest. Worse is a large, white, hot chocolate containing a whopping 719 calories and 33.4g of fat. Be wary of fast-food chains that make hot chocolates not with milk but with a mix of sugar and non-dairy creamer (containing the unhealthy partially hydrogenated soybean oil and more sugar).

How to make it healthier: Go for a small, no-whip, skinny hot chocolate to drop your calories to 209.

Vanilla Frappuccino

What is it?	A blended cream drink made from a coffee-free mix of sugar, syrup, milk and ice, possibly topped with whipped cream
Calories:	Small, 344; large, 530
Fat:	Small, 12.5g (7g saturated); large, 18g (9.9g saturated)
Verdict:	Blended creams are a mix of sugar, milk and ice and contain just 190 calories in a small cup. But, the addition

of syrups, such as banana and chocolate, turn them into a dieter's disaster. You'd be better off with a small pizza.

How to make it healthier: Skip the whipped cream to save 94 calories (131 in a large Frappuccino). Choose a small, low-fat coffee Frappuccino with no cream - just 119 calories.

Mocha

What is it?	Three-quarters steamed milk, 3-4 pumps of chocolate sauce and 2-3 shots of espresso topped with whipped cream
Calories:	Small, 255; large, 484
Fat: saturated)	Small, 9.3g (5.4g saturated); large, 25.3g (14.3g
Verdict:	Very fatty. This is sweetened with a massive 41g of sugar in a large cup. Things could be worse: a large white chocolate mocha with whipped cream contains 628 calories and 28.9g of fat

How to make it healthier: Order a small skinny (skimmed milk), no-whip (without cream) dark mocha and your calorie count drops to 175.

Drinking alcohol

It seems that in the western world we are having a major problem with alcohol. Our youngsters are falling into the streets drunk at the weekends and adults seem to be gulping wine down like there is no tomorrow. Because certain foundations say that drinking is good for you, especially red wine (I think they mean one small glass of red wine a day!) people are now using this as an excuse.

As part of this book I have researched the effects of alcohol on the body and it does not make pretty reading. It causes havoc with your liver and raises your blood sugar level, plus it is empty calories. I worked with somebody who drank an incredible amount and when she was dieting and stopped drinking her weight would drop by 10lbs in the first week as this was the water retention caused by the alcohol.

Also the wine glasses have got so much bigger that people are once again fooling themselves. A small pub measure of white wine is about 60-80 calories, making a bottle way over 600 calories – how many people do you know who drink a bottle of wine a day?

Alcohol makes you hungry so you eat more and combined with the empty calories and water retention it makes sense to drink as little as you possibly can. It also strips all the vitamins and minerals out of your body so this makes you unhealthy. It lowers your mood, makes you more stressed, tired and depressed – are you convinced yet?

Also a word of warning about cocktails – mixing all that alcohol together is not only lethal for your blood sugar and your health but it is also lethal for the calorie uptake as well!

Living to eat rather than eating to live – try to remember the calories!

In the 50s and 60s (especially after rationing in the war), few people ate out and most people had a sensible meal at home which was normally described as 'meat and two veg'.

With so many celebrity chefs cooking up amazing meals, plus the fact that most people eat out at least one a week, if not more, our culture has changed from eating to live to living to eat. I hear people discussing an up and coming meal in such detail, what they are going to have and how many courses but what they seem to forget is that it is very fattening.

Even though a lot of people don't talk about calories, you certainly have to take them into account somewhere along the line and if you are eating a three course meal that is laden with butter and cream, the calories will be sky high. Even an average pizza is about 2,000 calories which is, in my case, two days normal daily allowance when you add on your other food such as fruit.

Also, please remember that if you are adding a latte a day to your intake, even if it is a skinny one, you are still adding extra calories and you should make cuts elsewhere. I say this when I recommend that you eat a handful (small!) of nuts a couple of times a week – you cannot simply add another 150 calories a day to your diet without making a small cut somewhere else. If you are eating an extra 300 calories a week just by including a few nuts, then add the calories up for a year that will be a good few pounds added to your waistline!

When people go on holiday they seem to go mad. I watch people at breakfast and they must eat three times the amount that they would at home. Then it is pizza and chips for lunch and a three course meal with alcohol in the evening. Added to the fact that apart from a bit of swimming or walking they are really doing no exercise, this will turn to fat quite quickly. Why do they have to do this? In the sun with all that lovely colourful fruit and vegetables people should be eating healthier not worse food!

Celebrity chefs and cooking program and their fattening books!

We are now inundated with chefs and cooking program and books – they are on all the time bombarding us with food – most of it very unhealthy! It seems that grilling has given way to frying and although olive oil is good for you, you don't need that much and you certainly don't need it on every meal. They encourage three courses (which I have talked about before – YOU DO NOT NEED THIS MUCH FOOD!) so the calories in one sitting must be absolutely astronomical.

Now cakes and cup cakes are making a comeback - all that wheat and sugar and calories - everything that is bad for you in one mouthful!

Having spent 50 years trying to get people to grill food, now everyone is frying again. You don't need to fry anything and if you do you just need a spray of a low calorie oil. I never fry onions for soups, for instance, and I don't think it makes any difference to the taste.

So don't buy their books or make slimming adjustments – this is now recognized why lots of people are now putting on weight – but it is easily remedied but using slimming cook books! A word of warning as well that vegan and vegetarian cooking is not necessarily slimming so don't assume it is. It used a lot of cheese and beans have quite a few calories.

Electrolyte balance

The level of any electrolyte in the blood can become too high or too low. The main electrolytes in the blood are sodium, potassium, calcium, magnesium, chloride, phosphate, and carbonate. Most commonly, problems occur when the level of sodium, potassium, or calcium is abnormal. Often, electrolyte levels change when water levels in the body change. You then become either over hydrated or dehydrated.

For example, although I had lots of excess water in my tissues I was dehydrated and craved salt, showing an electrolyte balance. The balance can change for many reasons, especially the use of diuretics, laxatives and other medication.

Through this book I have talked about the problem with water retention causing weight gain, lack of minerals upsetting metabolism and being dehydrated causing hunger pains. If you feel that your electrolyte balance is not right please consult a qualified practitioner or doctor.

White fat cells and damaged brown fat cells

We have two types of fat cells which we affectionately call white and brown! The main functions of the brown cells are to burn fat to create energy and generate heat, therefore upping t your metabolism. On the other hand, white fat cells are the 'conventional' form of fat that we all recognize. They are designed to store energy for use in times of need. Chock full of lipid droplets, these big cells accumulate under the skin and around internal organs.

These fat cells (also known as adipose tissue) are considered to be part of the endocrine system and produce a lot of important hormones including leptin and estradiol (part of the oestrogen group).

Wouldn't it be great if we could turn white fat cells into brown fat cells? The good news is that scientists are already working on this one!

The bad news is that when your brown fat cells don't burn the fat and therefore don't boost the metabolism. This is now recognised as being one of the reasons for obesity.

You also need GLA (gammalinolenic acid) to activate the brown fat cells. However, you can get this from taking Omega 6 fish oils but make sure that you are not blocking production by a diet with a very high fat content, with butter and cream, for example.

Scientists in Kent are trying to develop a switch that will activate the brown fat cells – hurry up please!

Geopathic and environmental stress

Use of mobile phones, computers and sleeping near electricity can interrupt with normal functioning of the brain and the body. Also ley lines can cause problems, especially if they run underneath where you sit or sleep. These are quite easily overcome with devices that you stick on your phone/computer. For ley lines and geopathic stress I would recommend that you consult a practitioner for the best way to block the energy.

Thinking too hard

Canadian boffins discovered that we eat about 225 calories more after concentrating than relaxing, possibly due to our brain trying to refuel its energy tanks. So make sure if you are doing a lot of thinking to choose a healthy option, like a nut bar.

Irresistible!

Scientists have discovered why some people just can't resist food. Scans used to show the reward centres in some people's brains are particularly sensitive to food advertising and product packaging.

Researchers showed people pictures of highly appetising foods (eg cake and chocolate), bland food (eg broccoli) and disgusting food (eg rotten meat) and at the same time they measured brain activity with a MRI scanner. A questionnaire was then completed to assess their general desire to pursue rewarding items or goals. The results showed that the participant's scores on the reward sensitivity questionnaire predicted the extent to which the appetising food images activated their brain's reward network.

As people are constantly bombarded with images of appetising food items it is not surprising that obesity is on the increase. It is nothing to do with greed or lack of willpower but, in some people, an involuntary, exaggerated neuro-physical response to pictures of desirable food which, presented through clever advertising, makes it incredibly difficult for some individuals to resist.

Food manufacturers and advertisers must therefore take their share of the blame for obesity.

Resistance to losing weight

A study by researchers at Queensland University of Technology shows that the human body is designed to strongly resist losing weight. Dr Neil

King says that our bodies have strong mechanisms that defend attempts to lose weight but weak mechanisms that prevent weight gain. It is thought that evolution taught our bodies to resist dieting back in the days when food was scarce.

However, although I am no doctor I am not sure that I agree with this. Although I had trouble losing weight that was because my endocrine system and brain chemistry were completely shot. As I have mentioned before, if this is the case, how do celebrities lose weight and get down to a size 0?

You are not exercising or eating to suit your DNA

As well as different body types scientists are now showing that our individual DNA may need certain food and exercise – so you could be doing totally the wrong exercise for you and it could be hindering you rather than helping you. I have had a DNA test and it was fascinating and yes I made a few adjustments to what I was doing and it really helped. Research on the internet which company/test is best for you – and don't forget to look for money off vouchers before you buy as it can cut the cost by half!

A sucker for crisps

Scientists have found that we get a buzz from simply biting into crunchy foods. Experts say each bite creates both a clearly audible 'crunch' and a series of ultrasound waves that make the eating experience even better. The inaudible waves – generated at the sort of frequency that bats, whales and dolphins use for echo location – trigger a reaction in the brain which causes a pleasurable experience.

Professor Malcolm Povey, a Leeds University physicist, says that food is, in effect, talking to us and we innately understand what it is saying about textures by interpreting the sensations through our ears and mouths. His research shows that the sound and feel of food in the mouth is as important as taste, look and smell in deciding whether we like something or not. Apples topped the scale (healthy!) but followed by crisps and biscuits. The results showed that the foods rated as the tastiest also gave out the highest ultrasound readings.

I knew I liked crisps for a reason - I can blame it on that now!

Addiction

Scans of overweight people revealed the regions of the brain that controlled satiety were the same as those in drug addicts. If this is your problem, go straight to the amino acid section and see which supplements you need.

Addiction can also be genetic and that is when tools like EFT™ and self-hypnosis come into their own so you can reprogramme yourself.

Protection

I have mentioned this in my book several times but I want to mention it here as well. Your body can use fat as protection and it's not just by overeating. Your subconscious is clever enough to change the whole way your body works – never underestimate your subconscious! So no amount of dieting will get rid of excess body fat if it is serving an emotional function. You therefore need to look at every area of your life very carefully, both now and in your childhood. This protection is also very common in somebody who loses weight but always puts it back on again quickly.

In the olden days we were frightened of being starved to death, being eaten by some big creature or that we would freeze to death, so it is in built into our cells to add fat if we feel threatened in this way at all.

Some of the forms of protection are to do with making yourself unattractive because of relationship issues or previous sexual abuse. What better way to become sexually unattractive than to be obese? Also the body can put on excess weight as a way to reinforce feelings of inadequacy and of being unloved. It is like a self-fulfilling prophecy that feeds on itself. The worse I feel about myself, the fatter I became. The fatter I become, the worse I feel about myself and so it goes on.

I had a channelling with an ascended being and I was asking him about my weight and then we started to talk about how obesity was out of control and why this was happening. He came up with a very interesting story. He said people are putting layers of fat around themselves because they are frightened. They are frightened to go out because of the crime rate and muggings and murders. The television is always bombarding us with real time pictures of wars and killings that bring death and destruction straight into our living rooms – and it is frightening. You don't even feel safe in your own front room now. So their subconscious is layering them with fat to protect them – interesting, isn't it?

The body is now also layering fat to protect it against radiation waves from phones, tablets etc with which we are being bombarded all the time – this is even causing the death of the bees.

Fat is being placed round toxins in our body to protect the body – this is the subconscious's way of protecting the body but it is not very helpful and this fat will not come off until you address the toxin issue.

Fear of the lack of something

You may not know that you have this but quite a few of us have fear of the lack of something and it is normally brought into this life with us from past lives. This is where we died from starvation or poverty and we fear this will happen now. It may have also come from your parents who were broke and told you there wasn't enough money or food, or they never showed you enough love. It could be an ancestral pattern so it is a good idea to study your ancestors and see whether they had lack or whether they had enough food, money and love.

Lack will cause you to hang onto your weight as you fear that food is scarce. It puts you in a "poverty consciousness" as you are programmed with lack and can't release it. So if you earn money you might find yourself even making mistakes so you get sacked. You may find it very difficult to get your business off the ground or have the life you deserve.

This lack does not just concern food but also money; as the economy is not good at the moment, the fear could be triggered and you will start eating for no apparent reason. Also, as you can't hold onto or earn money if you are unemployed, the body will hold onto the fat as the only thing it can hold onto at the moment to help the lack.

I have excellent techniques to help clear this fear of lack, which is usually very deep seated and I have tremendous results.

Spiritual, mental and emotional starvation

Are you doing something that you don't want to do? Do you feel that you are missing something in your life? Do you know your life's purpose? Is your relationship unfulfilled? This could mean that you are literally being starved spiritually, mentally or emotionally and this could have a two-fold effect – you could start eating more to feed this starvation or your body could hold onto the weight.

You really need to look at your life – are you with the right person? Are you doing the job that makes your heart sing? Is there something you would like to do? If you are not doing what you want to do you will find that your overate or put on weight as compensation. You need to follow your heart or you will have an unhappy life and be overweight too boot!

Prader-Willi syndrome

PWS is caused by an abnormality on chromosome 15 which occurs around the time of conception and causes a variety of symptoms including obesity, poor muscle tone and an insatiable appetite.

There is a fantastic website at http://pwsa.co.uk/main.php which explains the genetic causes and gives help and support to sufferers and their families.

Older mothers

If your mother was older than average when you were born, it might account for you being overweight, so new research says. My mother was older (38, which in 1955 was considered a very old mother) and I was 12lbs when I was born. However, my husband, whose mother was reasonably young when she had him, was 12lb 12ozs, so I am not too sure about this theory!

Karma and past lives

I do talk a lot about weight issues coming from past lives and from karma but I do want to mention it again here. Ellen, from Heal Past Lives, believes that if you have 50lb or more to lose then it is likely to be a karmic issue or karma obesity as she calls it.

This karma can be anything from being starved to death in a past life or, like me, self-punishment for things done in previous lives. This would account for why people are becoming increasingly morbidly obese and, once again like me, whatever they do doesn't work. As I keep saying, it is not simply overeating but the body stops functioning correctly and the weight just piles on. This is also why people can lose the weight but then put it all back on again. As you know, my subconscious knew I could lose weight so filled me full of water instead.

If you are not into past lives or karma I still urge you to take this seriously. This book is all about being open to every possibility – and please remember that there are many people alive now who went through the holocaust in Germany and Russia and starved to death and this will still be in their cell memory.

You will have seen a lot of books, DVDs and emails about being able to manifest what you want, so you should be able to manifest a slim and healthy body! Unfortunately this isn't as easy as it seems, as all the thousands of people who bought the books are finding out. You have to heal all your issues before you can manifest and this is normally connected to karma.

Allergies

Allergies will put on weight – no doubt about it. For example, if you are sensitive to gluten (found in bread and pasta) it will give you the symptoms of an underactive thyroid. This also explains why thyroid tests can be so inaccurate. I have a huge section on allergies and intolerances and how to heal them.

An energy of desperation stops you in your tracks!

We all know that feeling of desperation when nothing works. But this energy will actually stop the weight loss as you are not connecting to your subconscious or your true self to allow it to happen. I know it is difficult but use EFT™ or meditate to overcome this but you need to be calm and still for the connection to work.

Unrealistic expectations

People (especially if they are dieting for the first time) get down to their correct weight but then it becomes difficult to sustain for all sorts of reasons. We have all seen the celebrities who lost the weight, did the exercise dvd and then put it all back on again! You cannot keep up three hours of exercise a day or 500 calories – your body wants to be nourished and cared for. Be realistic with your weight loss and stick with a figure that you can maintain easily.

Self sabotage

I am always banging on about this so I can't add it to the book too many times! As mentioned before I am the queen of self sabotage! I used to sabotage myself in an empty room! Do you find that a relationship is going well and then you pick fights? Do you find that a job is wonderful but then you make silly mistakes and your reputation goes down the pan? Do you start a diet and exercise routine and then find on day 5 you totally blow it? This is all your subconscious trying to stop you! In all honesty your subconscious does it because it thinks it is protecting you so don't get cross just heal all the reasons it is doing this with the techniques in this book.

If you get the inner critic telling you "you are going to fail" or "you are stupid", stop it in its tracks and tell it to go away – however strongly you want!!! You are succeeding!

Don't give up

Just because you have blown it for a day don't beat yourself and think you have blown it so you give your permission to keep blowing it!! Enjoy your day, dust yourself up and then go back to it tomorrow. You are not a bad person – you are human!!!

Programming

When you are born you are already full of programs. This could be soul programming or it could be from your karma or about the experiences you will have in this lifetime. Then you start being programmed by your parents, siblings, teachers, colleagues and everybody else! Not all these programs are for your highest good. You have to be a detective to sort through all of these programs and heal the ones that don't suit you now by using the techniques in this book.

Too restrictive

The moment you set yourself up on a restrictive routine (cabbage soup diet for example) you are setting yourself up for failure. Believe me I have been there! You can't keep up that up for life, perhaps a week or month but no longer. This is why it is best for you to develop your own eating plan for life including the things you like + masses of vegetables cooked in the way you love! This way you will stick to your plan and have fun at the same time.

And last but not least – POOR ME!

Poor me syndrome (also known as being a victim) is not an attractive quality so you need to snap out of it immediately!!! However you feel there is always somebody much worse off than you and at least you can do something about it! It is time now for you to take control of your life and your weight and crack it once and for all – no more excuses. No more blaming your family or your doctor as it won't help you.

I hear excuses all the time. "Ann it is so difficult for me to go out to eat because I am surrounded by food and people are trying to make me eat it" – rubbish I have been eating out for over 50 years and its fine! "Ann it is so difficult for me not to drink because people think I am odd and keep trying to force me to have one" – rubbish I haven't drunk for over 25 years and I don't have this! These are all excuses so stop making them otherwise you will be fat for the rest of your life and only have yourself to blame! Sorry to sound hard but its true – when I gave up a 40 a day habit (and I loved smoking more than anything else in the world) people used to say that it was so easy for me – why? It was because they couldn't do it. It was the hardest thing I had ever done but I was determined I was going to do it and only put on a 1lb.

Some people don't want to put any time or effort into something or they want somebody to do it for them – this doesn't work as you need to change. You have to make time in your diary to use the techniques in this book, do your exercises and plan your menus. Take responsibility now as the weight is not going to drop off on its own.

I won't work with clients now who are not willing to help themselves and want me to do it for them. If you don't change your attitude, your beliefs and become more positive it won't work.

SO NO MORE EXCUSES – LETS GET STARTED

Section 2

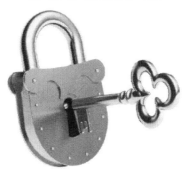

HOW BELIEFS, PATTERNS AND BLOCKS RULE YOUR LIFE

Chapter 4:

WHAT ARE BELIEFS, PATTERNS AND BLOCKS. HOW ARE THEY AFFECTING YOUR WEIGHT NOW?

What are beliefs and how are they affecting your weight now?

We are made up of our beliefs, some of which are negative and these can stop us moving forward and fulfilling our full potential which includes weight loss. These beliefs shape our lives and define who we are as people and if we try to step outside these beliefs we then sabotage ourselves so we end up back to where we started.

Are you confident? Do you believe fully that you can be successful and earn the money you deserve? Do you actually know how much you believe you are actually worth? Do you deserve the salary you think you do? Or do you believe that you are lacking in some way and this will affect your weight as you try and hold onto it. You might find that your subconscious mind and belief system are miles apart on this one.

Do you believe that you are not capable, inadequate, less than others and any other such beliefs? These beliefs are crippling your life and you will not move forward until they are replaced with a totally positive belief system so that you absolutely believe in yourself.

These beliefs can come from past lives, karma, ancestral karma and lineages, from programming when you were a child and by learnt behaviour as you have been growing up. Think about all the times you have been told that you have failed or were not good enough and these then become part of your belief system. When we are constantly told negatives about ourselves we believe them. At the moment there is a lot of talk about praising children too much so that when they do encounter a problem they totally collapse. But take my word for it, when you are constantly criticised and put down, it affects you very badly. So, as with everything else, moderation is the key.

What beliefs are holding onto your weight?
- I am inferior

- I am lacking
- I am inconsequential so I have to make myself big to be seen
- Losing weight is too difficult
- I will fail and put the weight all back on again
- I must be so awful and bad not to be able to control my eating
- I want to punish myself
- It is too hard to start dieting
- My weight is ancestral and I can't change that
- My weight is genetic and I can't change that
- I am not good enough/I am not enough
- I self-sabotage myself
- I am worthless
- I loathe myself

Healing negative beliefs

The best ways to heal negative beliefs and build confidence are:
- Emotional Freedom Technique (EFT™) – see chapter on EFT™
- Bach Flower Remedies
- Affirmations
- Ask your guides and angels to help heal you

Or book a session with me!

What are patterns and blocks and how are they affecting your weight now?

We all have patterns and blocks that affect us every day of our lives. These are part of our spiritual growth and they keep appearing until they are healed and dissolved – have you ever noticed that you keep attracting the same situation or the same harsh person? This is the universe showing you the patterns and blocks that need to be released. When you stand up to the aggressive person you will find that you don't encounter that type of person again.

A **pattern** is a program that you have which is part of your personality. For example, in your personality could be the thoughts:

- I am not good enough
- I am useless

- I can't lose weight
- I am not as good as other people
- I am stupid
- I am ugly
- I am fat (remember if you tell yourself you are fat you will be!)
- I am to blame
- It is my fault
- I can't do anything right
- I am a failure

This means that you block your weight loss as you feel that the task is too daunting and you will fail. New patterns can be easily installed using EFT™.

A **block** is something that stops you moving forward and the biggest one of these is FEAR. The other one is being safe. If your subconscious feels that it is not safe it WILL NOT LET YOU DO IT. So if your subconscious feels that losing weight is not safe, you WILL NOT LOSE WEIGHT!

Also, if you think you are worthless or you feel you do not deserve, this will cause you to self-sabotage.

Healing negative patterns and blocks

The best ways to heal negative patterns and blocks are:
- Emotional Freedom Technique
- Bach Flower Remedies
- Affirmations
- Meditation
- Ask your guides and angels to help heal you

Or book a session with me!

What is self-sabotage?

The term, self-sabotage, describes our often unconscious ability to stop ourselves being, doing or having; being the person we want to be, doing what we want to experience or achieve or having our goals and desires become reality. Most of the time we are totally unaware that we are self-sabotaging as it happens on a subconscious level. However sometimes we are aware of that little voice in the back of our head that says, "*you can't learn a language*" or "*don't be ridiculous you can't lose weight*".

Our subconscious mind is a powerful tool and always thinks that it is acting in our best interest. Stopping us stepping into new territory, discouraging us from taking risks ensures that we <u>don't</u> get hurt, we are <u>not</u> humiliated and we <u>don't</u> fail – that is why so many projects never get off the ground. Rather than playing to win, self-sabotage plays to avoid defeat.

The purpose of this aspect of the subconscious is self-protection and survival. It can even negatively affect your health if it thinks that this will protect you from a greater risk. Layers of excess weight have long been recognised as protection and very often the subconscious will use weight gain to protect you from perceived dangers you might be exposed to as a slimmer person. For example, where someone has been abused as a child, the subconscious may add weight to make them unattractive (it thinks) so that the abuse is never repeated.

So people may talk about self-sabotage in regard to their weight because they eat emotionally and put on weight. However sometimes self-sabotage will affect your hormones and/or organs, causing weight gain in people who eat only a modest amount. Sometimes people <u>can</u> lose weight but always put it back on: just another method of self-sabotage. Once the perceived need to protect through self-sabotage has been healed and released, our illnesses and weight may disappear.

My experience of self-sabotage

In my personal quest to lose the weight and water I had accumulated, I consulted a lady who specialised in 'muscle testing'. When we asked the question "Do I want to be slim", the clear reply was **"no!"** which took me totally by surprise. So then started the journey of discovery as to why my subconscious didn't want me to be slim.

Why was I self-sabotaging?

During the long seventeen years in which I slowly cleared and healed the reasons for my self- sabotage:

- I had set up a self-punishment/self-destruct program because of what I had done in past lives

- I had set up a protection around me (weight and water) because of the sexual abuse, date rape and male attention I had had – I didn't feel it was safe to be a woman
- I had several past life issues with starving to death and didn't want to starve in this lifetime
- I had several past life issues with dying of thirst, hence the excess water in this lifetime to ensure that it didn't happen again
- I had a tremendous amount of other karma
- I thought that if I became a therapist I could not trust myself not to hurt, or experiment on patients, as I had hurt them before in past lives and so I was only going to be a therapist when I was 'slim'
- I was frightened to take herbs as I had seen so many people die from them in past lives
- Because I had been persecuted in past lives for healing people, I thought I would be persecuted in this life as well
- I was frightened of being powerful
- I was frightened to do the work I was supposed to do
- I was frightened that the book would fail

Although I relate to my self-sabotage with weight and health there were many other areas of my life that affected.
- I was always in debt and could never pay off my credit cards
- I never got the job I deserved and was very often out of work
- If I got a job, there would always be someone giving me a tough time (karmic payback!)
- When I had any treatments, such as red vein treatment or plastic surgery, it would always go wrong

Believe it or not, my subconscious was creating the reality where all of the above occurred – the subconscious is that strong, believe me. Even when I had released the attachments, and got rid of the influence of my mother, my subconscious was still following their examples and as I strived to get better my subconscious really kicked in and made it worse.

So my subconscious was actually affecting all my organs and making them work inefficiently so that I put on six stone and swelled up with water. This was because my subconscious knew I could lose weight and it decided this was the best plan of attack.

That's why some people lose weight and then put it back on. The subconscious doesn't always realise what is happening to begin with, hence the weight loss. It then kicks in big time in survival mode and the weight goes back on. You would not lose six stone and then put it back on again – you might put back a stone and then get it off. People blame diets or losing it too quickly but, in fact, it is simply your subconscious sabotaging you.

Emotional and comfort eating

When you read magazine articles they always talk about emotional eating and weight gain. Some people do eat for emotional reasons and boredom. Some people do overeat and there are explanations for this. You need to identify your emotional eating triggers and use a technique such as EFT^{tm} to eliminate them. However, if you want to eat try to wait for a 10 minute period breathing deeply and you should find that after that the need to eat has gone.

However, I know a lot of slim people who overeat and drink too much. They overeat for emotional reasons as well – slim people aren't perfect or without their own problems.

One of the reasons I wrote this book is to show that overweight people do not eat emotionally any more than slim/normal people. How often are you on holiday and you watch people eat an enormous breakfast, followed by an enormous lunch and then three courses for dinner, plus booze, every day for two weeks? How often do you see a slim person eat a packet of biscuits or a bar of chocolate? ALL THE TIME!

You have to find the reasons why your subconscious doesn't want to lose weight and either release the reasons if these are past lives based or change your subconscious 'belief system' if they are more personality traits.

Removing the self-sabotage

When I was spending a huge amount of money with therapists and nothing worked, I did mention that I might be self-sabotaging myself. Most of them threw their hands up in horror and told me it was just an excuse to overeat (here we go again, I thought).

I read a lot about Emotional Freedom Technique (EFT™) and in the very first paragraph I read it mentioned self-sabotage. This was quite amazing. However, my self-sabotage was so deeply ingrained that for a long time EFT™ just made everything worse, as my subconscious tried to hold onto its control of me.

I therefore had to dig much deeper by clearing the attachments, past lives and karma and then I could use EFT™ and my other techniques to change my subconscious perception and its belief system that "I did not deserve".

Psychological reversal

This is a subject on which I talk in great detail in the chapter on EFT™ and is very important in the healing process. This is where you think you want to do something but your subconscious doesn't want you to - unfortunately your subconscious will win hands down every time!

I thought I wanted to lose weight but I actually didn't and my subconscious was stopping me. You need to find out all the reasons why and release and heal them one by one. For this you use the EFT™ psychological reversal techniques.

How are you self-sabotaging because my experience would lead me to believe that you are?

Habit of self-sabotage

I had a spiritual reading session and was told that the self-punishment had been healed but that I still had the 'habit' and that needed to be healed and not recreated. I feel it is very important to include it in this book, as it would have never occurred to me that I still had the habit and was capable of recreating the habit at any time. Our body and subconscious sabotage us so much that it becomes automatic and then a habit. So even when the original stimuli is healed the habit remains. So remember to test to see whether there is a habit and then heal accordingly (normally the same way you healed the original pattern). Make sure you don't recreate the habit by repeating affirmations and if you feel yourself slipping back into 'deserving the pattern' immediately cancel this feeling and ensure that you keep healing it.

What is secondary gain?

Believe it or not, every illness and problem can have a significant benefit for the person who is experiencing it. Professionals uses the term 'secondary gain' for this well known phenomenon and you will start to recognize this behaviour in people that you know. In some cases, the benefits of having the problem are so great they outweigh the suffering the problem is causing.

This problem is created by the subconscious, totally unbeknown to the person. Often this person is pushing themselves too hard and the unconscious mind will come up with a way to deal with what is going on in that person's life so an illness or a problem is created that is not under their control.

A good question to ask yourself is "what are the benefits to you that this illness or the problem bring and why are you keeping it around?". So what are the benefits of you holding onto the excess weight? Analyse this question very carefully and dig until you get to the bottom of it.

Some examples of secondary gain:
- You have hurt your leg but it stops you doing something you don't like and you get lots of sympathy – a double whammy!
- You put on weight and this stops you going out of the house and your entire family are worried about you and fuss over you
- A friend looks after a relative and is always rushing around after them. All her friends tell her how marvellous and dedicated she is so she in turn gets lots of attention and sympathy that she wouldn't get if she stopped

Do you recognise yourself here?

Watch your thoughts!
Watch your thoughts, for they become your words;
Watch your words, for they become your actions;
Watch your actions, for they become your habits;
Watch your habits, for they become your character;
Watch your character, for it becomes your destiny.

Your subconscious believes everything it hears!

Remember that your subconscious listens to what is said to you by other people or yourself and it takes everything it hears literally. It cannot differentiate between a joke and reality, so never put yourself down, even as a joke. So, if you keep telling yourself that you are FAT your subconscious will make you fat and keep you that way. Your fat cells will think – I am fat so I better keep my cells nicely plumped up and not lose them. Yes, this is really true!

I know it sounds amusing but this is what happens in real life and the wonderful poem displayed at the top of the page becomes your reality – and what you **believe** becomes your **truth**.

We talk about beliefs a lot in this book and changing them from being negative to positive – so we are looking at positive thinking here. The half full glass rather than the half empty glass.

I was told I was fat, stupid and ugly from the first moment I remember and therefore that is what I believed. Even when I lost weight, I still believed I was fat and because I projected that outwards other people treated as if I were still fat too. Now when I look at pictures of myself as a plump child or a slim adult, I think that actually I am beautiful; perhaps a little large but certainly not fat, stupid or ugly.

Once when I was on holiday there was a little Italian girl on the beach – she was quite plain. All the adults around her kept calling her beautiful and clever and she had such a smile which showed that she believed it. This belief would follow her into adulthood and she would believe that she was beautiful, slim and clever for the rest of her life and I think this is absolutely brilliant! I thought how wonderful of these people to instill such fabulous qualities in one so young. In our day we were never good enough, never lived up to expectations – were a disappointment. Never were we told that our parents loved us and I still know people to this day who are trying to get their parents approval – even though they are over fifty.

I will never say anything negative to anyone, let alone someone young – they are always beautiful, great and clever and I am always proud of them – I wish someone had told me that they were proud of me.

Talking about yourself

So you must talk about yourself with positive beliefs, even if you don't believe them at the time – fake it until you make it (as is the current phrase!) and in the case of weight problems, think like a slim person. A friend of mine who had put on a lot of weight said that she was surprised when she saw a picture of herself at that time, as she believed she was still slim – so it does work both ways!

Most people who are overweight are normally very critical and always speak negatively about themselves. They normally suffer from low self-worth and low self-esteem. The result is that, by doing this, they are perpetuating the problem. When you are speaking negatively to yourself, ask yourself if you would speak to a friend like that. The answer most probably will be that you wouldn't, so why on earth are you speaking like that to yourself? Stop it now!

It is almost impossible for your body to change when you keep sending it negative messages. As long as you say, "I am FAT," you give your body more instruction and energy to BE FAT.

You need to change your chatter from negative to positive even if you don't believe what you are saying. I hear you cry "How can I be positive when I am fat?" but it is very important in the re-programming of your subconscious and your cells. Positive affirmations are an excellent way of re-programming and these can be combined with EFT™ for stronger and quicker results.

Change 'I am fat' to 'I am getting slimmer every day'

Change 'I never lose weight' to 'It gets easier every day to lose weight'

Changing beliefs

People ask how they can change their beliefs and luckily these days there is a variety of techniques and therapies to help do this but you also have to be careful not to fall back into any bad habits.

This relates to all areas in your life and not just to weight, so let me tell you a couple of stories:

I love Sunday nights as this is my pamper night where I have a long bath, face mask and do my nails. Some of my friends hate Sunday night because they have to go back to work on Monday and they don't like their jobs. I have changed my perception of Sunday night so that I enjoy it, unlike my friends who dread it.

When I was made redundant I opened up my own beauty salon, thinking that this was the best job in the world and something that I had always wanted to do. In reality, it was long hours for very little money, putting up with bolshie people who treated my staff and myself appallingly. This taught me to love whatever job I was doing because there is no magic job that you will love for eight hours a day – each one has its ups and downs. Therefore I changed my perception.

Other Therapies

Other therapies and techniques that are good for working on and changing the belief system are:

- EFT™
- Affirmations/Afformations
- Hypnosis and Self Hypnosis
- NLP

Accepting who you are and loving yourself

If you despise your body you get into a downward spiral of low self-esteem and self-loathing. You need to accept how you are now and be happy - remember that losing weight doesn't necessarily mean you are going to be any happier than you are now. Acceptance is also surrender and you give up the fight – once you have done this you will find your angels and guides can give you more help.

Love your body and thank it for all it is doing for you at this moment. Your body is doing an excellent job and it needs to be appreciated and thanked. You have to start changing your perception of yourself and I know only too well that this is not easy.

Start loving yourself. This is not an ego love but a self-worth love and you are worthy. For some unknown reason it is very difficult to look at yourself in the mirror and say "I love you" but this is important. Everybody has their unique traits, so write down yours and repeat them several times a day. If you don't love yourself and keep putting yourself down you are opening up the path for everybody to treat you the same way.

EFT™ always incorporates "I love and accept myself". Sometimes people find this difficult to say but after using EFT™ for a while you realize that you are wonderful and that you love and respect yourself.

Cancelling negative statements

Remember, if you say something negative, immediately say "CANCEL THAT LAST STATEMENT" – you can say it out loud (if you have made the comment) or under your breath if someone else has made a negative statement. If it helps, wear an elastic band around your wrist and ping it every time you make a negative statement – it stings and really stops you! It is very important to remember this technique as very often we say things all the time which are habit, such 'I am sorry'. If you want to apologise, say "I apologise" as this has a very different energy to I am sorry.

These are positive statements to say after cancelling a negative statement:

- 'I am healthy and well nourished'
- 'I love myself, I love my body and my excess fat disappears'
- 'I am my ideal weight'
- 'I enjoy exercising several times a week'
- 'I can say 'no''
- 'My body is nourished'
- 'I am proud of my body'
- 'My metabolism works at 100%'
- 'I am spiritually, emotionally and physically balanced'

Affirmations and Afformations

In personal development, an **affirmation** is a form of autosuggestion in which a statement of a desirable intention is repeated in order to implant it in the mind. An **afformation** is the same but it is asked as a question because the subconscious loves questions and finds ways to answer them.

Louise Hay who wrote *You can heal your life*, advocates affirmations for every area in life from health to work to home. Louise Hay believes that we cause our illnesses and with the use of affirmations we can begin the self-healing process.

Louise Hay's explanation for Bell's palsy is 'total unspoken rage'. When I was aged 20 my parents were moving house and insisted that I went with them. I tried very hard to refuse but was soon cowed by my mother who insisted that I would be 'out on the streets' if I didn't move with them. The morning of the move I woke up with severe Bell's palsy. I ended up having an operation which involved shaving off most of my hair and cutting off my ear in order for the surgeon to scrape the nerve causing the palsy. This, in fact, put me more into the clutches of my mother as I had an incredibly crooked face for two years and no hair! When I read 'total unspoken rage' I knew that was exactly how I felt. From that moment on I realised that we did cause our own illnesses, we just had to realise it.

I think everyone needs a copy of Louise Hay's books for reference as she talks about how to phrase the affirmations and how often to repeat them. You must always repeat an affirmation at least three times at once and this set must then be repeated several times during the day. Remember it is REPEPITION that you need but do not include more than three positives in one statement. When I was doing a replacement I wanted to put:

'I am beautiful, slim, fit, healthy, wealthy and successful'

But with my teacher, we changed it to:

'I am slim, healthy and fit'

Remember that affirmations should be positive. I knew someone who started to affirm to himself, "I am not hungry." He actually gained weight. Each time he told himself he was not hungry he focused his attention inside to see if he was hungry. He thought about hunger so often that he put conscious energy into being hungry. He was hungrier when he used an affirmation denying hunger than when he didn't think about hunger. He should have said something like "I am feeling slimmer every day" or "I am totally nourished".

The subconscious also strips out the word NOT so it should never be in an affirmation statement. Using the example above, 'I am not hungry' becomes 'I am hungry' – another reason for weight gain.

If you give yourself a negative message, do the following:
- Stop and ping your elastic band
- Say CANCEL that last statement immediately
- Immediately repeat a positive affirmation three times

To work, affirmations should be in your own words and must feel real to you. You need to say them out loud in a strong voice and really feel them and mean them. Here are a few examples of affirmations that you could use – if you wish to use an afformation, just say it as a question, for example 'Why am I so healthy?'

If you feel you are going to cheat:
- 'I'm losing weight now'
- 'I love the feeling of making progress'

To keep you on the straight and narrow:
- 'I'm getting fitter every day'
- 'I am feeling thinner today'
- 'I am getting slimmer and slimmer every day'
- 'I'm losing weight now'
- 'I look and feel lighter today'
- 'I'm enjoying how I'm feeling now'
- 'I love the feeling of making progress'
- 'I love the food that makes me thin'
- 'I am going to fit into the next size smaller any minute'
- 'I enjoy being healthy'
- 'My body is getting stronger, slimmer, and healthier every day'
- 'I feel so thin inside, my outer is just about to catch up'
- 'My metabolism is burning up all the food I eat'
- 'My weight will stay stable for the rest of my life'
- 'I am powerful'

Saying affirmations quickly
Recently a therapist told me of a brilliant way to get the most out of repeating your affirmations. If you are like me you will have rakes of them, ranging from money to weight to career to health and every time you repeat them it becomes such a mouthful. So type your affirmations up and give them a number. I then say "Affirmation 1 will be xxxxx" and then repeat this affirmation three times. This affirmation then becomes 'Affirmation 1', or '1' in my subconscious.

In future, instead of having to repeat all the affirmation say 'Affirmation 1', 'Affirmation 2' etc. They really roll off your tongue and you can ensure that you get multiple repetitions done very quickly and efficiently!

Absorbing the affirmations quickly
As you are repeating your affirmation, tap around your scalp just outside and around your right ear (this is called temporal tapping). This

helps absorb the affirmations into your brain more quickly than just saying them.

Switchwords

Switchwords were first identified by Freud and then researched by James T. Mangan in the 1960s. These power words **speak directly to our subconscious mind**, helping clear blocks to success and activating our ability to manifest health and weight loss, love, money, self-healing and success.

How do Switchwords differ from Affirmations? An affirmation reprograms the subconscious with positive thoughts as the affirmation is chanted continuously for many days. It is quite hard to reprogram the subconscious as if it doesn't believe the affirmation, it will put up blocks and may sabotage the new belief. It is like chanting an affirmation saying "I am rich and wealthy" – the subconscious is more likely to say "No you are not!" and it won't allow itself to be reprogrammed.

A Switchword talks directly to the subconscious and it automatically activates it – the subconscious understands what it is saying, loves it and allows itself to be activated. The Switchwords may not make sense to you (especially the phrases) but it makes perfect sense to the subconscious. The subconscious will then allow itself to be "reprogrammed" and release all blocks and sabotage to it happening. Switchwords can be used in conjunction with EFT and can be chanted any time of the day. Try to chant at least 10 times in one set and then do at least 3 sets per day. If you prefer to write the Switchwords down this is fine as well.

Switchwords for weight loss:
- To get figure back: RESTORE-BE
- To forgive yourself and feel safe when you have lost weight (and trust yourself): FOREGIVE-RESTORE
- Angel number for weight loss – DIVINE-555
- Frequencies for weight loss – DIVINE-295.8 HERTZ
- To remove resistance: RELEASE-RESISTANCE
- To cut calories – CUT
- To cut down eating and habit of eating - DIMINISH-CUT-BE-GUIDE-POINT
- To want to lose weight – DIVINE-CHANGE

Section 3

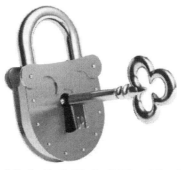

WHAT IN YOUR BODY IS CAUSING WEIGHT GAIN?

Chapter 5:
DIFFERENT BODY TYPES AND THEIR EFFECTS ON YOUR WEIGHT

Genetics and build

When you look around at the population you see that people come in innumerable different shapes and sizes. This is partly due to genetics but also to do with build. Some builds can lose weight (or even have trouble putting on weight) and some builds put on weight just looking at food. This is not an illusion, this is the truth!

When I first started to research diets and exercise, I came across a very useful book written by Dr Sandra Cabot on different body types. From her research she then added another body type and this shows how much experience she has with body types and how she understands them. I have looked at other explanations of the three main body types, but I liked Dr Cabot's explanation and description of them all, including her new one, so I decided to incorporate her research. Dr Cabot very graciously gave her permission for me to use her work in this book. Dr Cabot also recommends diet and exercise to suit your body shape.

I highly recommend Dr abot's website and books as she is not only a diet expert but an expert on liver and hormones as well. I suggest you sign up for her newsletter, as it is packed with useful information. Dr Cabot's website and books are listed in the Recommended Reading aapendix.

Although I use Dr Cabot's explanation of body types, I also list Ayurvedic and Chinese body types are well. You will see that they overlap and if your intuition points you in the direction of one of these other types, find yourself a good practitioner!

Body Frames

Also to be taken into consideration is the body frame – we have all seen people with tiny wrists and ankles and others who are more largely built. So how much you weigh will depend on your frame as well as shape etc. Also I know this sounds funny (but you must be used to this by now!) but I think that some people's bones weigh more than others –

I have been the same size as friends but I weigh sometimes more than 2 stone more – so this is my answer to that!

Female Wrist Measurements:

	Height less than 5' 2" (Less than 155cms)	**Height 5' 2" - 5' 5"** (155cms - 163cms)	**Height more than 5' 5"** (More than 163cms)
Small	Less than 5.5" (140mm)	Less than 6.0" (152mm)	Less than 6.25" (159mm)
Medium	5.5" - 5.75" (140 - 146mm)	6" - 6.25" (152 159mms)	6.25" - 6.5" (159 - 165mm)
Large	More than 5.75" (146mm)	More than 6.25" (159mm)	More than 6.5" (165mm)

Male Wrist Measurements

	Height more than 5' 5" (More than 163cms)
Small	5.5" - 6.5" (140 - 165mm)
Medium	6.5" - 7.5" (165 - 191mm)
Large	More than 7.5" (191mm)

In the past

Years ago it was recognised that there were different body types and they were categorised according to their shape only. This was before we understood the hormonal and metabolic differences between the body types. Sorry, Guys, if the explanation is a bit biased to the ladies but the descriptions still stand for the well-known types of body shapes, mesomorph, ectomorph and endomorph.

- Android was called the mesomorph
- Thyroid was called the ectomorph
- Lymphatic was called the endomorph
- Gynaeoid - this body type has not been previously described as it has been developed by Dr Cabot – it has never been identified before because it is mainly a woman's hormonal body type and is probably a combination of several other body types.

Dr Cabot's information on Your Body Type and Weight

There are four classic body shapes or body types; they are the –
   Android Body Type – apple shape
   Gynaeoid Body Type – pear shape
   Thyroid Body Type – long and skinny all over shape
   Lymphatic Body Types – round and puffy all over shape

The different body types are classified according to the anatomical proportions of their bones and where they store fat.

Each body type has unique hormonal and metabolic characteristics, which explains why some body types gain weight easily and are more prone to cellulite. Your body type also determines the areas of your body where excess fat will accumulate.

The vast majority of people will belong to one of these four body types. Around 10% of people are a combination of two body types. The body types are genetically determined so you will probably find someone in your own family with the same body type as yourself. Your body type determines your metabolic type and is important to know because it explains the foods that may cause problems for you. When you avoid the foods that are incompatible with your body type, weight loss becomes much easier.

Android Body Type

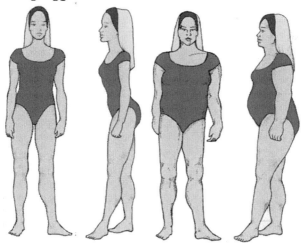

Android ideal   *Android overweight*

Approximately 40% of women and the vast majority of men belong to this body type. It is characterized by broad shoulders, strong muscular arms and legs, a narrow pelvis and narrow hips. The waistline does not curve inwards very much, so the trunk has a somewhat straight up and down appearance. Android women have a boyish figure, and are usually good at sports and are athletic and strong.

Android-shaped people have an anabolic metabolism, which leads to a body building tendency in the upper part of the body. Weight gain occurs in the upper part of the body and on the front of the abdomen, so that an apple-shape may develop.

Android Body Type Weight Control Tablets contain the herbs Red Clover, Dong Quai and Milk Thistle and the liver nutrients choline and inositol and the fiber chitosan.

Gynaeoid Body Type

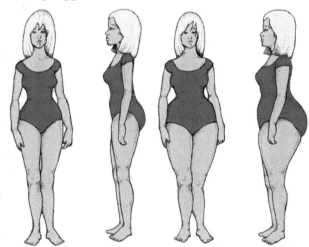

Gynaeoid ideal   **Gynaeoid overweight**

Approximately 40% of women belong to this body type, which is characterized by small to medium shoulders, a narrow tapering waistline and wide hips. Weight gain tends to occur on the buttocks and thighs, which accentuates the pear shape of the Gynaeoid type. The hips and thighs curve outwards and excess weight gain occurs below the waistline. Gynaeoid women are "estrogen dominant", which means that the hormone estrogen has the greatest influence in their body shape.

They often have a relative deficiency of the other female hormone called progesterone. Excessive estrogen promotes fat deposition and cellulite around the hips, thighs and buttocks. Natural progesterone balances the effect of estrogen and helps to reduce weight from the hips and thighs.

The Gynaeoid body type is uncommon in men, however very occasionally you will find a man who falls into this category.

Gynaeoid Body Type Weight Control Tablets contain the herbs Wild Yam, Parsley Piert, Vitex Agnes Castus, Gymnema Sylvestre and chromium picolinate to assist their weight loss.

Thyroid Body Type

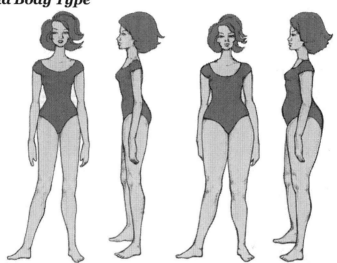

Thyroid ideal   **Thyroid overweight**

Approximately 10% of women and 5% of men belong to this body type, which is characterized by a fine (small) bone structure, relatively long limbs compared to the trunk and a long narrow neck. Thyroid shaped people often become dancers or fashion models, and can be described as having a 'race-horse' or 'grey-hound' appearance.

Thyroid types have a high metabolic rate and do not have as many fat cells as the other body types, which means that they do not gain weight easily; thus they can often eat much larger amounts than their friends without showing the effects. We call them thyroid types because they have such a rapid and efficient metabolism, and not because they are more likely to suffer with thyroid diseases.

Interestingly thyroid women are often naughty with their diet, in that they miss meals and live on stimulants, such as caffeine, diet sodas, fizzy soft drinks, sugar and cigarettes.

Blood sugar imbalances often result from the overuse of stimulants, which may lead to fatigue, but thyroid types try to overcome this with more stimulants!

They do not put on weight easily because they do not build muscle easily and they do not store fat. They have a smaller number of fat cells than the other body types so there are not many places on their body where they can store fat. They often try to put on weight as they feel too skinny. If they become very underweight, especially in combination with smoking and a deficiency of nutrients, their estrogen levels may become very low. Low estrogen levels lead to a reversible loss of breast tissue and feminine curves, and in the long term osteoporosis.

Thyroid Body Type Weight Control Tablets contain the minerals chromium picolinate, magnesium and zinc combined with glutamine, vitamin B 5 and the herbs Liquorice and Ginseng to balance their metabolism.

Lymphatic Body Type

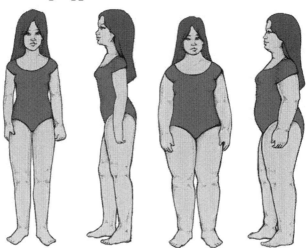

Lymphatic ideal   Lymphatic overweight

Approximately 10% of women and 5% of men belong to this body type, which is characterized by weight gain all over the body.

The limbs have a thick puffy or spongy appearance and the bone structure is not very visible. There is a layer of fat and fluid all over the body, which is excessively thick. These people have often been plagued with weight excess since childhood. Lymphatic people have a very slow metabolic rate, which causes them to gain weight very easily. They also have an inefficient lymphatic system, which leads to fluid retention and makes lymphatic people appear fatter than they really are. Cellulite is common in this body type, with deposits of fat swollen with lymphatic fluid, giving a dimpled appearance on thick puffy limbs.

Lymphatic types may have imbalances in pituitary hormones, such as prolactin and growth hormone mediators, and overall they are hypersensitive to hormones.

Lymphatic Body Type Weight Control Tablets contain the herbs Fenugreek, Celery, Horseradish and Fennel combined with kelp, cayenne, rutin, selenium and vitamin B 6 to assist with weight loss.

> *To discover your Body Type now visit www.liverdoctor.com and do the interactive questionnaire on line – get your answer now!*

The Apple Shape versus the Pear Shape

Apple shaped people accumulate excess weight in the trunk and inside the abdominal cavity and on the abdominal wall.

People who carry excess fat around the abdomen are at an increased risk of diabetes and heart disease. These people are commonly Android or Lymphatic Body Types and are more resistant to insulin than those who store most of their body fat in the hips and thighs. The latter are known as pear shaped or Gynaeoid Body Types. According to Dr Cynthia Sites from the Vermont College of Medicine, "efforts to reduce either subcutaneous abdominal fat or intra-abdominal fat should be helpful in reducing the risk of type 2 diabetes in post menopausal women". Their study found that the higher the abdominal fat stores were, the less the body was able to respond to insulin.

How do you know if you are apple shaped?

Measure your waist and hips with a tape measure while unclothed. To do this measure your waist one inch (2.5cms) above the navel, or at its narrowest part, while standing with the abdominal muscles relaxed. If there is no smallest area around the waist, take the measurement at the level of the navel. Then measure your hips at their widest point while standing.

Divide your waist measurement by your hip measurement to get your waist to hip ratio.

A waist to hip ratio of over 0.8 for women, and over 1.0 for men is suggestive of an unfavorable accumulation of fat around the middle, which increases diabetes and heart disease risk.

Ayurvedic Body Types

As I am talking about body types, I thought I would add in the body types relevant to Indian Medicine, called Ayurvedic. You will notice that they match up with the three main body types once again reinforcing that your body type is instrumental in how you manage your weight and exercise. Again most people are normally a comination of two types but one type is normally predominant.

This is what an Ayurvedic practitioner would recommend for each body type for food, exercise and herbs balance the body.

Remedies	Vata	Pitta	Kapha
Food	Warm, well cooked food. Sweet, sour and salty tastes	Warm to cool rather than steaming hot. Sweet, bitter and astringent tastes.	Decreased quantities of warm food. Pungent, bitter and astringent tastes. To be taken earlier than 10 am and not later than 6pm.

Exercise	Moderate exercise such as yoga, walking and light weights	Moderate exercise which may include jogging, swimming, Yoga, cycling and weight lifting	Regular and vigorous.
Herbal Dietary supplements	Ashwagandha, shatavari, haritaki, Guggul, Trikatu, Vata tea, Calming Tea.	Haritaki, Bhumiamla, Chyavanprash, surakta, sitopladi churan, pitta Tea.	Guggul, sitopladi churan, trikatu, chyavanprash, Kapha Tea

Vata body type (ectomorph)

Here are some of the common characteristics of people who have a predominantly Vata constitution.

- Creativity, mental quickness
- Slenderness; lightest of the three body types
- Tendency toward cold hands and feet, discomfort in cold climates
- Excitable, lively, fun personality
- Variable appetite and digestive efficiency
- Physical Features:

People of vata constitution are generally physically underdeveloped. Their chests are flat and their veins and muscle tendons are visible, the skin is cold, rough, dry and cracked. Vata people generally are either too tall or too short, with thin frames which reveal prominent joints and bone-ends because of poor muscle development.

Physiologically, the appetite and digestion are variable. Vata people love sweet, sour and salty tastes and like hot drinks. The production of urine is scanty and the faeces are dry, hard and small in quantity. They have a tendency to perspire less than other constitutional types. Their sleep may be disturbed and they will sleep less than the other types. Their hands and feet are often cold.

Pitta (mesomorph)

Here are some of the common characteristics of people who have a predominantly pitta body type.

- Medium physique, strong, well-built
- Strong digestion, strong appetite; get irritated if they have to miss or wait for a meal
- Mind is focused and sharp
- Tend toward anger, frustration or irritability when under stress
- Excellent memory

Physical Features:

These people are of medium height, are slender and body frame may be delicate. Their chests are not as flat as those of vata people and they show a medium prominence of veins and muscle tendons. The bones are not as prominent as in the vata individual. Muscle development is moderate.

Physiologically, these people have a strong metabolism, good digestion and resulting strong appetites. The person of pitta constitution usually takes large quantities of food and liquid. Pitta types have a natural craving for sweet, bitter and astringent tastes and enjoy cold drinks.

Kapha (endomorph)

Here are some of the common characteristics of people who have a predominantly Kapha constitution.

- Easy-going, relaxed, slow-paced
- Physically strong and with a sturdy, heavier build
- Slow moving and graceful
- Tend towards being overweight; may also suffer from sluggish digestion therefore not losing any weight

Physical Features:

People of kapha constitution have well-developed bodies. There is, however, a strong tendency for these individuals to carry excess weight. Their chests are expanded and broad. The veins and tendons of kapha people are not obvious because of their thick skin and their muscle development is good. The bones are not prominent.

Physiologically, kapha people have regular appetites. Due to a slow metabolism and a poor digestion, they tend to consume less food but cannot lose weight.

Chinese Medicine

A very simple explanation of Chinese Medicine is that it is based around the five elements, Water, Fire, Wood, Earth and Metal which aren't exactly different body types but all of these elements refer to different parts of the body and control how they work. Chinese medicine has been used over 5,000 years with great success and if you would like to know what element you are I would suggest that you select a local practitioner or buy a book and get the good old dowser out!

Chinese doctors then prescribe herbs and diet according to what type of element you are. Again you are likely to be a mixture of two and once you understand the concept you can see how this affects your health, weight and build – it is really fascinating.

From a weight loss point of view the one with which I have had great experience is water, as this is the one that controls the kidneys and bladder. When being diagnosed I was informed I was mainly water with a little fire that gave me damp! The diagnosis was correct because obviously I have suffered with tremendous water retention, my kidneys and bladder have not worked correctly and I like my food cooked – apparently raw food makes damp worse. Also I was informed that I shouldn't drink too much water as it added to my problem – something I had suspected for a long time.

Conclusion

During various chapters in this book I have discussed how everybody is different and how everybody's health and eating needs will also be different. Even if you have genes that contribute you being overweight it doesn't mean that you can't overcome them.

In the chapter on Eating for Life, I have already talked about the metabolic and blood group diets and in this chapter we have looked at different body types from the view of an Australian doctor, an Indian doctor and a Chinese doctor.

Because all the body types are different and all like different foods and metabolise them differently, you have to be so careful when people make blank statements like:

✓ You must eat your food raw
✓ You must eat your food lightly steamed
✓ You must eat 5 meals a day
✓ You must drink 1½ litres per day

For example, if I were to drink 1½ litres a day it would literally flood me and sink to my legs making them rock hard. If I were to eat five meals a day, however small, I would certainly put on weight. I also find raw food very hard to digest and it adds more damp to my existing damp, as the Chinese doctor informed me!

As I keep harping on about in this book, everybody is different and must do what is right for them. You need to find out exactly what type you are and then put together your unique plan for life. This is where using a diagnostic tool is handy as it removes all the guess work.

Remember, DIETS DON'T WORK!!

Chapter 6:
THE ORGANS THAT CAN BE RESPONSIBLE FOR WEIGHT GAIN

I have thought long and hard about how to write this chapter. I eventually decided to keep it short, sweet and in layman terms but with the added benefit of all the fixes that can be applied to each organ. If you want to know more about the organs and how they all interact with each other, there is a massive amount of information on the internet which explains the organ functions much better than I ever could.

Some of my comments are made from experience rather than appearing in a medical text book – doctors may not agree with me but that's fine. We always have our diagnostic tools to fall back on to check out any anomalies and I have lived this – the doctors haven't.

Louise Hay is a marvellous lady who has several books based around affirmations. The book *'You can heal your life'* shows what emotions are causing the organs to fail and what affirmations you should say to heal those problems.

Louise Hay says that fat is needed for protection and that is why some of us surround ourselves with fat even though we don't know against what we need to protect ourselves. Louise's affirmation for this is 'I am at peace with my own feelings. I am safe where I am. I love and approve of myself'. All affirmations should be said at least three times at one go and then repeated as often during the day as you can manage.

Louise Hay's affirmations are listed under the relevant organs. The only organ she doesn't cover is the hypothalamus.

Although in this book I talk a lot about an underactive thyroid, I am also talking about all the organs that can stop you losing weight as I firmly believe that they are all interlinked – especially to the hypothalamus. I also don't mention cholesterol as I believe there is a lot of hype about this and as long as you are eating healthily, I believe it is best not to take medication. Al Sears gives a lot of advice about lowering cholesterol naturally and claims that the medical profession have it totally wrong. My husband was on statins and he is still suffering the consequences now – he was depressed, suicidal, foul tempered, his personality totally changed, he had joint pains that moved around his body and they gave him stomach problems. Even though he has been off them for years he is still suffering with the joint pains. If you want to lower your cholesterol use the yoghurts, spreads and other alternatives that are available. Al Sears also gives lots of advice about high blood pressure which I make sure that Don follows to the letter.

Endocrine System

As I will say many times in this book, the body is such a finely tuned instrument it is surprising that it works at all. The endocrine system is fantastically complicated, with all organs inter-relating and between them covering nearly all the metabolic processes of the body.

If any of your endocrine organs don't work properly (with the exception of an overactive thyroid) you certainly will not lose weight and, in most cases, you will put it on and have that 'out of control' feeling that I talk about in Chapter 2, 'My Story'.

The major glands that make up the endocrine system are the hypothalamus, pituitary, thyroid, parathyroid, adrenals, pineal and the reproductive glands, which include the ovaries and testes. The pancreas is also part of this hormone-secreting system, even though it is also associated with the digestive system because it also produces and secretes digestive enzymes.

The endocrine system relates to all the chakras which are covered in more detail in the chapter on how to use crystals to help lose and maintain your weight.

All the related herbs, homeopathy, vitamin, minerals and eating plans are covered in their respective chapters. However, I do add to the sections anything that I think is vital for that organ's recovery, especially if I have had experience of it.

Hypothalamus

The hypothalamus is a collection of specialised cells that is located in the lower central part of the brain and is the primary link between the endocrine and nervous systems. Nerve cells in the hypothalamus control the pituitary, thyroid, adrenals and pineal gland by producing chemicals that either stimulate or suppress hormone secretions. More information is being discovered about the hypothalamus all the time and now it is recognised that it controls the water balance in the body as well.

Leptin, which resides in all fat cells, communicates directly with the hypothalamus in the brain, providing information about how much energy is currently stored in the body's fat cells. For example, when fat cells decrease in size, leptin decreases, sending a message to the hypothalamus to direct the body to eat more. Contrariwise, when fat cells increase in size, leptin increases and the message sent to the hypothalamus is to instruct the body to eat less. Research is now proving that it is not as simple as the explanation here but most are agreed that leptin levels have dropped due to the advice of recent years to eat a diet mainly of carbohydrates. Eating protein on a regular basis can help raise leptin levels and there are plenty of herbs that are listed in the appropriate chapter that will help. Personally I don't have a problem with leptin as I don't have a large appetite, but understand how frustrating it is when you are never full and always want food.

There are excellent books available on the subject of leptin and what to eat which are listed in the Suggested Reading section of this book. A couple of supplements say that they help with leptin:
- Slim Factors with Leptin from Supplements to go
- Liporex from from Liporex-leptin-solution
- LeptiBurn from Biotrust

Grehlin is secreted by the stomach and plays a major role in appetite regulation so I have included it under this section. It is referred to as the 'hormone of hunger': however, when obese individuals lose weight, this often results in an elevation of grehlin, also promoting food intake, and thus may be a physiological reason why there is difficulty in maintaining the new found weight with dieters.

People who fail to sleep properly over-stimulate their ghrelin production which increases the desire for food. Simultaneously, lack of sleep reduces the production of leptin which will make you hungry. It has been found that thinner people have higher levels of ghrelin production during certain night time hours which is lacking in people who suffer obesity. In addition, it appears that food does not suppress grehlin levels in obese individuals, again contributing to overeating. I know this doesn't relate to the hypothalamus but as it helps control appetite, I thought I would slip it in here. I am also investigating other ways of controlling your appetite if you have a grehlin problem as there is not much information available as yet.

Grehlin also decreases metabolism and the ability to burn brown fat.

Yo-Yo dieting – researchers in Spain have discovered that those who gained back their weight had higher levels of leptin and lower levels of ghrelin.

Why a gastric band may help other than just cut down on food

During the procedure, the size of the stomach is reduced and some of the upper intestines are bypassed. It is thought that the ghrelin hormone may normally be produced in the bypassed areas of the gastric system. Dr. Edward Lin, the lead researcher in the study, believes that ghrelin is one of the most powerful appetite stimulating hormones naturally produced in the body. Lowered levels of the hormone may help patients lose weight after their surgery, along with the strict post-surgical diet and the smaller stomach.

Another study conducted by doctors at King's College London and Hammersmith Hospital discovered that gastric bypass patients produced higher levels of the PYY hormone. This hormone is normally released after a meal to tell the brain you're full. After a meal, most thin people's PYY hormone level increases by 50%. However, the study found that post-gastric bypass patients had a 150% increase in their levels of this appetite suppressing hormone.

Interestingly, obese patients who did not undergo the weight loss surgery had little or no increase in the PYY hormone after a full meal. Also, the increased hormone level was found in patients after standard gastric bypass surgery, but not after a gastric banding.

Research is now underway to see if these hormonal changes may be used as an alternative treatment for obesity, without the surgery. Hope for a non-surgical weight loss cure was stirred in 2002 when researchers reported some success in reducing the weight of obese rats with the PYY hormone. Unfortunately, other researchers have been unable to repeat their findings.

My comments:

I believe that this gland also has a hand in controlling the levels of the neurotransmitters and amino acids that we talk about in the section on brain chemistry. The hypothalamus also controls the body's temperature clock and the hunger mechanism which includes releasing and controlling leptin and grehlin. I also believe that it feeds the thyroid, the pituitary, adrenals and the pineal with vital hormones as well.

There is no medical help if your hypothalamus doesn't work – if fact, most doctors would not recognise that it doesn't work but, believe me, if this gland is slightly out of balance it can cause you tremendous problems.

Alternative therapies:

Homeopathy	Hypothalamus extract (either homeopathy or supplement form)
Australian flower remedy	Bush Fuscia
Karma and past life work	The hypothalamus is a very old gland so therefore if you have a problem now the cause may be due to karma and/or past life work. This is always a good place to start. Once cleared and working properly, you normally find that it enhances your healing powers
Diet	Protein and fat with a little carbohydrate
Vitamins	All required
Minerals	All required
Chakra	No specific chakra as 'belongs to whole'
Other	Access to sunlight as often as possible

Pituitary

Although it is no bigger than a pea, the pituitary gland, located at the base of the brain just beneath the hypothalamus, is considered the most important part of the endocrine system. It's often called the 'master gland' because it makes hormones that control several other endocrine glands. The production and secretion of pituitary hormones can be influenced by factors such as emotions and seasonal changes. To accomplish this, the hypothalamus relays information sensed by the brain (such as environmental temperature, light exposure patterns, and feelings) to the pituitary.

The pituitary is divided into two parts: the anterior lobe and the posterior lobe. The anterior lobe regulates the activity of the thyroid, adrenals, and reproductive glands. Among the hormones it produces are:

- growth hormone, which stimulates the growth of bone and other body tissues and plays a role in the body's handling of nutrients and minerals – this could also cause fat calves and ankles
- prolactin which activates milk production in women who are breastfeeding
- thyrotropin which stimulates the thyroid gland to produce thyroid hormones
- corticotropin which stimulates the adrenal gland to produce certain hormones
- ACTH (adrenocorticotrophic hormone) which stimulates the production of hormones from the adrenal glands
- TSH (thyroid-stimulating hormone) which stimulates the production of hormones from the thyroid gland
- FSH (follicle-stimulating hormone) and LH (leuteinising hormone)

The pituitary also secretes endorphins, chemicals that act on the nervous system to reduce sensitivity to pain. In addition, the pituitary secretes hormones that signal the ovaries and testes to make sex hormones. The pituitary gland also controls ovulation and the menstrual cycle in women – so this is the organ that was responsible for me having three weeks' PMS a month!

The posterior lobe of the pituitary releases an anti-diuretic hormone, which helps control body water balance through its effect on the kidneys and urine output and oxytocin which triggers the contractions of the uterus that occur during labour.

My comments:

Wow, you can see how important the pituitary is for all over body functioning, let alone weight loss. If this little baby doesn't work properly you are in big trouble!

The only medication a doctor will give you for any problems or imbalances in the pituitary is limited and in my experience doesn't help with weight loss.

Alternative therapies:

Homeopathy	This is individual but there are combinations available
Herbs	Siberian ginseng, vitex (chasteberry), tribulus, gotu kola
Australian Flower Remedy	Yellow Cowslip Orchard
Pituitary	Either as homeopathy or supplement
Karma and past life work	As with the hypothalamus, the pituitary is a very old gland so therefore if you have a problem now the cause may be due to karma and/or past lives
Diet	Protein and fat with a little carbohydrate
Vitamins	All required
Minerals	All required
Supplements	Growth hormone can be purchased in many forms
Louise Hay	Louise Hay says that it represents the control centre therefore the affirmation should be "My mind and body are in perfect balance. I control my thoughts".

Chakra	Brow/Third eye
Other	Access to sunlight as often as possible
Other Reasons	Traumatic childbirth can cause problems with the pituitary and the thyroid. You may have a tumour which is normally non-cancerous

The Pineal

The pineal gland is located in the middle of the brain. It secretes melatonin, a hormone that may help regulate the wake-sleep cycle and is instrumental in Season Affective Disorder (SAD) where you are happy in the summer but sad in the winter. SAD causes weight gain and depression and encourages you to hibernate all winter.

My comments:

I believe that the pineal is under rated and has many more functions than doctors currently think. Twenty years ago, doctors thought that the pineal had no function at all. I have suffered from SAD for years and this was instrumental in me putting on a stone over the winter months. I was one of the first of everyone I know to buy a light box, which I found effective to a certain extent. However, you need to sit in front of a light box for several hours a day, preferably in the morning, which makes it impractical to use. Also research now shows that sitting in front of a light box can damage your eyesight so you do have to be careful.

Other alternatives:

Homeopathy	Hypericum
Herbs	St Johns Wort, Gotu Kola
Australian Flower Remedy	Bush Iris
Pineal extract	Either as homeopathy or as a supplement
Serotonin or other amino acids	Light box which you use in the morning to emulate light rays
Vitamins	All

Minerals	All
Supplements	Melatonin
Diet	Can crave carbohydrates so try to eat regularly and not skip meals. Protein and fat are required for good organ function
Chakra	Crown/Third Eye

The Thyroid and Parathyroid

The thyroid, located in the front part of the lower neck, is shaped like a butterfly and produces the thyroid hormones thyroxin and triiodothyronine. These hormones control the rate at which cells burn fuels from food to produce energy so is the main controller of the metabolism and instrumental in weight loss. The production and release of thyroid hormones is controlled by thyrotropin which is secreted by the pituitary gland.

The hormone T4 circulates in the bloodstream but needs converting into T3 (by various enzyme processes). So if you don't have enough T3, T4 (which is called thyroxin) will not be able to perform the metabolic processes and you will put on weight. This is known as Wilson's syndrome and there is an excellent website and book that explains exactly what this is. There is also a condition called Reverse T3 which means that T3 will show up as fine in the thyroid test, but actually it doesn't work!

In the United States you can get T3 therapy but you are not offered it in the UK. Research is now being conducted into T0, T1 and T2 and how they affect the body and weight loss/gain – it is still in its infant stage at the moment but watch this space as I believe this information will help as to why thyroxin doesn't always help.

Attached to the thyroid are four tiny glands that function together called the parathyroids. They release parathyroid hormone, which regulates the level of calcium in the blood with the help of calcitonin that is produced in the thyroid.

There are many diseases of the thyroid gland including underactive (hypo) and overactive (hyper) – in this book we are only concerned with hypothyroidism. We mention Wilson's syndrome above, Hashimoto's Disease (with is an autoimmune problem) and there is thyroid cancer. When you have a thyroid problem you live on your adrenals to give you energy. This wears them out so as part of the thyroid treatment you should address your adrenal problem otherwise you may find that the remedies may not be as effective as they could be.

The thyroid is one of the organs that is most susceptible to the Epstein Barr Virus and this will most probably not be picked up by your doctor. I would suggest you buy the book, The Medical Medium as he gives you lots of advice on how to heal it. I would highly recommend Spirulina which is one of the best combinations of vitamins to heal a virus and the homeopathic remedy, Thuja at 200c strength. Please also contact me as I can remove virus's totally and heal the damage they have caused. It may take a couple of months but it is worth continuing with to feel better and lose weight.

My comments:
This is the most important gland for weight loss as it controls the metabolism and must be functioning correctly otherwise you don't stand a chance! Doctors and slimming clubs talk about this as if it was a rare condition but believe me it is as common as one in four people – no wonder obesity is rising!

The tests for under functioning thyroid are next to useless and when diagnosed in the UK the only medication given is Thyroxin – I have only known a couple of people with a metabolism-thyroid problem lose weight when on Thyroxin – and I know plenty of people with under active thyroids! This is because they have a good metabolism before they have a thyroid problem. They do not test in the UK for T3, so you could prove positive for T4 and will be given the results of not having an underactive thyroid when you do. Also whilst I am moaning about the NHS thyroid test I would like to point out that if you are just below or on the lowest scale, you will still be diagnosed as not having an under-active thyroid – how do they know that you don't need to be at the top of the scale?

Also when you have a thyroid problem, especially Wilson's Syndrome, your body temperature is normally slightly lower than normal. Check your temperature and relate that to your practitioner.

Metabolism:

Most doctors talk about the thyroid as controlling the metabolism and although I am sure that it plays its part, I am firmly of the belief that there are other hormones and processes that also control the metabolism and the Hypothalamus is one of them.

For example, in my studies I have noticed that if a person had a good metabolism before they developed an under active thyroid, that when they started to take thyroxin they lost all the additional weight. However, if you always had a slow metabolism (or a weight problem that hasn't come on suddenly), taking Thyroxin or straightforward thyroid homeopathy doesn't make the slightest bit of difference – a couple of the additional symptoms may go away but the weight stays firmly attached to your hips!

Other symptoms of an under-active thyroid are:
- Extreme fatigue
- Hair loss and thinning hair, no underarm hair
- Weight gain
- Water retention
- Dizzy when standing
- No sweating even when you should
- PMS problems and menopausal problems
- Inability to lose weight whatever you do
- After exercise muscle tone is not maintained
- Brittle nails, coarse hair and dry skin
- Anxiety and depression
- Puffy eyes and face and general oedema
- No half-moon on nails
- Hair, eyebrow and eyelashes falling out
- Hoarseness, sore throats, swollen tongue and not liking anything tied around your neck, such a scarf
- Skin tags
- Carpel tunnel syndrome
- Blocked nose, sinus and catarrh
- Tarsal tunnel syndrome (tingly and sore feet)
- No interest in food or never full and always hungry
- Fibromyalgia
- Bra bulge fat
- Loss of smell and taste

- Muscle and joint pain
and many, many more

Other alternatives:

Homeopathy	This will be different for every person
Herbs	Especially don't forget Kelp, Bladderwrack, Fucus, Spirulina and Black Walnut
Australian Flower Remedy	Old Man Banksia
Thyroid	Supplement (either as homeopathy, sarcode or a supplement)
Diet	Protein and fat with little carbohydrate. Protein, especially animal protein, stimulates the thyroid. The thyroid also needs fats to function. Food containing iodine is very important as the thyroid needs iodine for all its functions (which could be kelp and seaweed)
Louise Hay	Humiliation, not speaking your truth and not being able to stand up for yourself. Your affirmation will be "I move beyond my old limitations and now allow myself to express freely and creatively" and "I create a new life with new rules that totally support me"
SRT	SRT practitioners believe that this organ fails when you believe that God has abandoned you, either in this life or a previous one
Minerals	All but especially iodine and selenium. Don't overdose on iodine as it may stop the thyroid producing its own iodine
Vitamins	Lack of vitamins and minerals can be a significant reason why the thyroid doesn't work properly - All but especially B vitamins

Amino acid	Thyroid hormone is basically the amino acid tyrosine with some iodines attached. But I take a multiple amino acid – see chapter on amino acids for further information
Supplements	T-Convert from Nutri and other Thyroid support supplements especially from Dr Wilson
Fats	Omega 3 and especially Coconut Oil
Don't eat	Foods that degrade the thyroid:
	Cabbage, cauliflower, kohl rabi, sprouts, kale, swede, turnip, mustard, sweet corn – these should all be cooked.
	millet sometimes ; wheat sometimes – wheat can affect the thyroid function; lentils and kidney beans; soya products; peanuts. Avoid anything else that reduces the uptake of iodine by the thyroid
	Intolerance to wheat can cause a normal working thyroid to show signs of being underactive
Medication for the thyroid	In the UK, Thyroxin
Medication that can degrade the workings of the thyroid	Lithium (psychiatric illness), phenyl-butazone (ankylosing spondylitis), tolbutamide (diabetes), salicylates (pain), androgens (male sex hormones), sulphonamides (anti-bacterial), chlorpromazine (tranquilisers), phenytoin (epilepsy), levodopa (Parkinson's), steroids
Other Reasons	Sometimes childbirth and the menopause can cause a problem with the pituitary and the thyroid. Shock and stress – such as a death or being made redundant - can cause the thyroid to stop working.

Whiplash injury, having any operations in the region of the neck or having major dental work which has caused a misalignment of the jaw, which in turn results in a disturbed thyroid function. Also toxicity from dental materials such as amalgam and root canal fillings. Fluoride is now being shown to be one of the main reasons for weight problems at the moment. We need to have this taken out of our water. At one time our bread was supplemented with iodine and since this has been removed, thyroid issues have been on the rise.

Other organs	If the other endocrine organs don't work then chances are your thyroid won't. But please remember the adrenals – when you have a low thyroid you live on your adrenals to keep you going and they become exhausted. So to balance your thyroid you must also balance your adrenals. This is where a lot of doctors and natropaths make a mistake – they treat the thyroid but don't look at any other organs. That is why Thyroxin is not successful in many cases.
Karma and past life work	Look at all lives where you have starved to death or where you have been hanged or similar as this relates to the throat chakra. Weight can also be to punish you so look at those lives as well
This life	Look at either punishing yourself or protecting yourself due to sexual abuse or equivalent. Not being able to speak up for yourself.
Chakra	Throat

Adrenal glands

The body has two triangular adrenal glands, one on top of each kidney. The adrenal glands have two parts, each of which produces a set of hormones and has a different function. The outer part, the adrenal cortex, produces hormones called corticosteroids that influence or regulate salt and water balance in the body, the body's response to stress, metabolism, the immune system, and sexual development and function. The inner part, the adrenal medulla, produces catecholamines, such as epinephrine. Also called adrenaline, epinephrine increases blood pressure and heart rate when the body experiences stress.

This is one of the organs that is normally exhausted or overstimulated. Stress is one of the main causes of over stimulating the adrenal glands. Either way can cause weight gain, as will be explained in this section. Sometimes people with underactive thyroid glands will appear to be hyperactive – that is because their adrenal glands are pumped up for action and are literally keeping them going. But then the adrenals get exhausted which displays further symptoms. This is what happened to me and I nearly collapsed with adrenal failure.

Overactive adrenal glands:
Apart from diseases shown above, people can release excess cortisol to deal with stressful situations – that is why people are now saying that stress makes us fat.

Excess cortisol increases body fat levels, blood sugar levels and blood pressure. When we are under chronic stress the cortisol levels circulating in your body are elevated and this acts as a potent signal to the brain to increase appetite and cravings for certain foods, especially for carbohydrates and fats. Cortisol then acts as a signal to our fat cells to hold on to as much fat as they can and to release as little fat as possible. If that wasn't bad enough, cortisol then slows the body's metabolic rate by blocking the effects of many of our most important metabolic hormones including insulin (so you crave carbohydrates), serotonin (so you are low and depressed) and the growth hormone (so you lose muscle and gain fat).

Recently, I have had a very stressful experience and a mass of cortisol was released into my system. My hair started to fall out at an alarming rate, my finger tips were so sensitive that I couldn't pick up anything hot, I couldn't stop eating and I put on water around my middle that I couldn't get rid of. I experienced this increase in cortisol first hand.

If that isn't bad enough, research now shows that the stress of dieting could make us even fatter by making it harder for us to lose weight and easier for us to regain the weight we did lose.

Symptoms of over activity of the adrenal glands:
- Layer of fat around the middle but slim arms and legs
- Increase in the overall amount of body fat
- Water retention including moon face
- Reduced levels of weight losing hormones
- Increased blood sugar level

Symptoms of underactive or exhausted adrenal glands:
- Low blood pressure
- Allergies to certain foods
- Poor tolerance of heat and cold
- Frequent and constant thirst
- Weak appetite but cravings for sugar/sweet and salt
- Meal related bloating
- Chronic fatigue
- Light headiness and feeling dizzy
- PMS with hot flushes
- Linked with hypothyroidism and hypoglycemia
- Hypopituitarism (low hormones released by pituitary gland)
- Low thyroid function so you are 'living off your adrenals'
- Does not tolerate T3 therapy very well
- Not sweating as much as you should
- Can cause hot sweats

My comments:
Stress and the adrenals is one of the main reasons that people are putting on weight (especially round the middle) and not being able to lose it once it is there. You can see how important the adrenals are to good health and weight loss – especially with our busy lives and how the body reacts and copes. You need to follow the section on Other Alternatives very carefully, as you must have some form of stress release and relaxation every day.

Stress is addictive and it can be hard to get off the band wagon but you can. I have said before in this book that I think stress is a very over used word. People get stressed going to the supermarket or running the kids to school. Ten years ago you would have said that it was a pain or a chore. I have just recently finished a computer contract where I had to drive at least one and a half hours each way, sometimes two hours. I see accidents all the time and sit in long queues of traffic, so I could quite legitimately say I was stressed but I don't. I do my relaxation, I play with my dogs and I eat a healthy diet (and no alcohol!) and I am not stressed. You must do this to relax and not put you're your body and adrenals under pressure. With all the techniques for elevating stress you must do something about it now otherwise it will have very serious consequences.

Other alternatives:

Some form of relaxation	Meditation, CDs, yoga
Some form of exercise to release stress	Running, lifting weights, walking
Australian Flower Remedy	There would be different ones for different problems
Herbs	Liquorice is good (but not if you have high blood pressure). Ginseng has beneficial effects
Adrenal extract	Either as homeopathy or a supplement
Diet	Eat frequently, little alcohol and carbohydrates. Stop drinking caffeine
Louise Hay	Defeatism, no longer caring for self, anxiety. Your affirmation will be "I love and approve of myself" and "it is safe for me to care for myself"
Vitamins	All but especially A, B complex and C
Minerals	All, especially magnesium, manganese, chromium, copper, zinc and calcium
Supplements	Q-10, Omega 3, Siberian Ginseng
Others	Use Himalayan salt (www.mercola.com)
Chakra	Base

Explanation of hormones released by the Adrenals:

Cortisol: Cortisol mobilises and increases amino acids (the building blocks of protein in the blood and liver) and then stimulates the liver to convert amino acids to glucose, the primary fuel for energy production. It mobilises and increases fatty acids in the blood (from fat cells) to be used as fuel for energy production. It maintains mood and emotional stability and counteracts inflammation and allergies. Cortisol can cause fat around the middle and the "muffin top" when this causes stress.

DHEA: DHEA has many functions but the one in which I am particularly interested is that it decreases the percentage of body fat and increases muscle mass. It also improves resistance against viruses, bacteria, parasites, allergies, cancer and candida.

More importantly, it is involved in the thyroid glands conversion of the less active T4 to the more active T3 – something that I talk a lot about in this book.

On another note it reverses many of the unfavourable effects of excess cortisol, creating improvement in energy, sleep, PMS and mental clarity and accelerates recovery from any kind of acute stress.

Pregnenolone: Pregnenolone is a steroidal hormone manufactured in the body and is principally synthesised in the adrenals. Apart from helping with weight loss, well-being and ageing it is found to be one hundred times more effective for memory enhancement that other steroids – I must give some to my husband!

Balancing your meals for blood sugar control:

To maintain proper adrenal function it is imperative to control your blood sugar levels. An excessive ratio of carbohydrates to protein results in excess secretion of insulin that often leads to intervals of hypoglycaemia. The body, in an attempt to normalise blocked sugar, initiates a counter-regulatory process during which the adrenals are stimulated to secrete increased levels of cortisol and adrenaline. It follows that an excessive secretion of carbohydrates often leads to excessive secretion of cortisol. This contributes to chronic cortisol depletion and consequently adrenal exhaustion.

In order to stabilise blood sugar you must maintain a balance between two hormones, glucagon and insulin. Protein in the diet induces the production of glucagons and carbohydrates in the diet induce the production of insulin. Insulin promotes fat (energy) storage and when excess carbohydrates are eaten the body produces large quantities of insulin and little glucagons. This high level of insulin results in MORE FAT BEING FORMED AND STORED. Upper back fat and love handles are also associated with excess insulin.

The optimal level of insulin to glucagons is achieved by a diet that contains carbohydrates balanced with proteins in a ratio of approximately two to one (two grams of carbohydrate per gram of protein and gram of fat per meal or snack.

A small amount of fat or cold pressed vegetable or seed oil should be part of each meal in order to help control the rate of entry of glucose (blood sugar) in the bloodstream.

Herb	Effect	Contraindication	Dose
Magnolia Bark	Controls cortisol and has a general affect as an anti-anxiety and anti-stress agent	Too much could cause sedation and drowsiness	200-800 mg
Beta-sitosterol	Balances ratio of cortisol to DHEA		30-300 mg
Theanine	Controls mental and physical performance during stressful events		25-250 mg
Phos-phatidlyserine	Has a direct cortisol lowering effect		50-100mg
Aconite	Calms the body down		200c

Sex Organs

The gonads are the main source of sex hormones. In males, they are located in the scrotum. Male gonads, or testes, secrete hormones called androgens, the most important of which is testosterone. These hormones regulate body changes associated with sexual development.

The female gonads, the ovaries, are located in the pelvis. They produce eggs and secrete the female hormones oestrogen and progesterone. Oestrogen is involved in the development of female sexual features and both oestrogen and progesterone are also involved in pregnancy and the regulation of the menstrual cycle. Problems happen when you have too much oestrogen and become what they call oestrogen dependant – this is normally when you get water retention and PMT symptoms.

Fat on the arms is linked to low testosterone levels (I didn't know that I must admit). Fat around the hips, bottom and thighs is linked to excess oestrogen.

My comments:
I have a whole section relating to hormones as I believe that they prove to be one of the main weight gain issues that women have and hormones affect our entire monthly lives. Men are so lucky! However, low cases of testosterone in both men and women can cause a low sex drive and less muscle definition.

Homeopathy	Many to choose from but need to dowse to find correct one
Herbs	Lots of herbs to choose from that will have beneficial effects
Oestrogen extract	Either as homeopathy or a supplement
Diet	May crave carbohydrates, so don't skip meals – eat protein and carbs at every meal
Karma and past life work	Look at all lives where you have been sexually, physically or mentally abused or raped. Look at lives that have given you the belief you don't want to be a woman or a man
This life	You could be protecting yourself due to sexual abuse or equivalent. You could feel it is not safe to be a woman

Louise Hay	Affirm "I am completely safe as a woman"
Vitamins	All but especially B complex
Minerals	All but especially magnesium
Chakra	Solar plexus

Pancreas

The pancreas produces (in addition to others) two important hormones, insulin and glucagons. They work together to maintain a steady level of glucose, or sugar in the blood and to keep the body supplied with fuel to produce and maintain stores of energy.

Type 1 diabetes is when the pancreas fails to produce enough insulin. Symptoms include excessive thirst, hunger, urination, weight loss in some cases and tremendous weight gain in others

Type 2 diabetes is when the body can't produce normal amounts of insulin, in Type 2 diabetes the body is unable to respond to insulin normally. Children and teens with the condition tend to be overweight and it is believed that excess body fat plays a role in the insulin resistance that characterises the disease. Doctors, including Al Sears and Joe Mercola offer masses of advice on how to overcome this with diet and supplements

Syndrome X is the precursor to Type 2 diabetes and can normally be corrected by diet and supplements. The incidence of Syndrome X is increasing alarmingly and one of the reasons is a diet that includes refined flour and sugar, too many carbohydrates with too little protein, plus junk food, fizzy drinks and fried foods.

My comments:
One of the reasons that obesity is on the rise is that at least one in three people has Syndrome X. As our diets have been high in refined carbohydrates and fizzy drinks, with very little protein, we have been insulin resistant and we are starting to see this very strongly in our children as well. There is a wealth of research on the internet about insulin and how it causes weight gain: this is an important factor and one that is sweeping the western world. As usual, Al Sears and Joe Mercola are good places to start.

Other alternatives:

Homeopathy	Iris versicolor, Belladonna
Herbs	Gymnema Sylvestre, dandelion, olive leaf
Pancreas extract	Either as homeopathy or a supplement
Diet	Should get advice from a nutritionist for which ever condition you have
Louise Hay	Pancreas relates to rejection, anger and frustration because life seems to have lost its sweetness. Your affirmation will be "I love and approve of myself and I alone create sweetness and joy in my life"
Vitamins	All
Minerals	All
Chakra	Some say solar plexus, some say root

Liver

If your liver doesn't work correctly you will not be able to lose weight and may be toxic as it can't release the waste properly. Instead of me going through all the functions of the liver in great detail, I would highly recommend the webs site www.theliverdoctor which explains every function of the liver and what to do about it very simply and in a fun way. Sandra Cabot, who owns the site, is one of my heroes and she has a newsletter to which you can subscribe to get up to date information.

The liver is the largest organ in the body and is located in the upper right side of the abdomen. A simple synopsis is that it acts as a filter to remove toxins (harmful substances) and waste products from the blood. A healthy liver filters blood at a rate of about 1.5 quarts per minute. That's 540 gallons of blood a day and more than 13 million gallons over a lifetime!

The liver also stores nutrients such as certain vitamins, minerals, and iron, and plays a role in synthesising and managing levels of certain chemicals and proteins in the body, such as cholesterol, hormones, and sugars and it helps the body digest food.

So when you drink too much or eat fish and chips which are laden with fat, please give a thought to your poor old liver because it has to go into overdrive to break it all down and get rid of it. When you feel 'liverish' remember that your liver is trying to tell you something!

My Comments:
The liver is a forgotten about organ that has many important functions and you need to treat it with kindness and love, Sandra Cabot suggests lots of remedies on her site and I list below the ones that I know are extremely good.

Alternatives:

Herbs	Milk thistle is especially good and should be taken every day by everyone
Liver extract	Homeopathy or supplement
Tonic	A general liver tonic would be beneficial
Detox	There are various methods available on the internet for detoxing your liver – get your dowser out to see which one is best for you
Metals	Detox to get rid of excess metals
Parasites	Get rid of parasites – black walnut is the best remedy I have found and it also speeds up the metabolism at the same time
Louise Hay	The Liver is the seat of anger and primitive emotions. Your affirmation will therefore be "Love and peace are what I know" Use EFT™ or TAT to release any anger that you may have
Other Supplements	Use probiotics (kefir being the best one) and enzymes

Digestive Organs

All of your digestive system must be in full working condition for the nutrients to be absorbed and the waste to be expelled. I have combined the colons, the bowel and the stomach into one group to make it easier.

If you are constipated do not eat lots of carbohydrates such as rice, white pasta and bread because they will bung you up further You do need to increase your water intake – I found that red grapes and prune juice really helped me. Also if you use EFT every day for constipation you will find this disappears.

Another tip is do not drink when you are eating, especially water, as this dilutes the acid in your stomach and interferes with digestion. Drink half an hour before or after eating – I know this is terribly difficult. However, if you had one glass of wine, the acid would aid digestion.

My comment:
It is important to ensure that you don't have parasites and that you do have enough enzymes for digestion to take place. A lot of people recommend you eat raw food as this is easier to digest but I must confess that I like my food cooked. I feel that I digest cooked food better so it is back to your diagnostic skills to ascertain which is right for you.

Once you have adopted the correct eating plan for you, got your body balanced and eliminated your food intolerances you should find that your digestion really perks up.

Other alternatives:

Herbs	Especially Ginger, oregano oil, grapefruit seed extract, golden seal
Organ extracts	Homeopathy or supplement
Detox	There are various methods available on the internet for detoxing digestive organs – get your dowser out to see which one is best for you! Also do a colon cleanse before you do any other cleanse or detox, especially of the liver.
Metals	Get rid of excess metals

Parasites	Get rid of parasites – black walnut is the best I have found and it also speeds up the metabolism at the same time
Louise Hay	All these organs relate to fear of letting go of the old. Your affirmation will be "I freely and easily release the old and joyously welcome the new"
Other therapies	Use EFT to release constipation, IBS or any other complaint you have
Minerals	All, especially zinc
Vitamins	All, especially vitamin B
Other supplements	Use probiotics (kefir), digestive enzymes, gastrointestinal repair nutrients (glutamine and aloe vera), Omega 3
Allergies	Eliminate using EFT™ or chose to avoid the foods such as dairy, wheat, yeast etc.

Kidneys and Bladder

Your kidneys and bladder are essential for eliminating excess water and toxins through the urine. If these two organs are not working you will start to get oedema which is virtually impossible to get rid of once it has taken hold as the water sinks in between the cells which in turn slows all the processes down. These organs are very often overlooked when you have a weight or water retention problem but it could be the water that is causing the weight problem.

My Comments:
As you know from reading my story, my kidneys and bladder were the main trigger points of my self-sabotage so whenever I did anything that was 'good' for me, they would literally stop working and I would swell up with water. My ankles sometimes would swell up by at least 4 inches a day with great lumps around my once tiny feet and ankles. My legs were rock solid with no movement in them at all. If I showed a doctor

this the reply would be "that's fine – there is nothing wrong here". How on earth could that be? People used to say to me to continue using the herb or homeopathy that had triggered it in the first place and work through the pain! Well, I'd like to see them continue taking something when their kidneys have stopped working, the pain is intense and they are swelling up like a balloon! Talk is cheap in my opinion and most people offer the most ridiculous advice. Until somebody has something they have no idea what is happening or how it feels.

Other alternatives:

Homeopathy	Kali Phos, Cantharis
Herbs	Dandelion, uva ursi, cranberry
Kidney and Bladder extract	Homeopathy or supplement
Detox	For kidneys and bladder
Parasites	Eliminate parasites using black walnut
Other supplements	Cranberry juice (in small amounts) is excellent
Louise Hay	Kidneys relate to criticism, disappointment, failure and shame. Therefore your affirmation will be "Only good comes from each experience" Bladder relates to anxiety, holding onto old ideas, fear of letting go and being pissed off (we can all relate to that one!). Therefore your affirmation will be "I comfortably and easily release the old and welcome the new into my life" and "I am safe".
Vitamins	All
Minerals	All
Other hints	Drink mineral water throughout the day, sipping it but don't overdo it

Lymphatic System

The lymphatic system is a complex system, composed of organs, lymph nodes, lymph ducts, and lymph vessels that transport lymph from tissues to the blood stream. Lymph is a transparent fluid containing white blood cells, known as lymphocytes, and antibodies that destroy foreign substances in the body and are a major part of the body's immune system. Lymph vessels make up a network that covers every inch of your skin and surrounds each organ.

My comments:
When you have a thyroid problem, a sluggish lymphatic system seems to go hand and hand with it. To eliminate the waste and ensure that the lymph keeps on the move it is important to keep this system moving. One of the best ways of doing this is with a lymphatic drainage massage which is a special massage designed specifically for the lymph nodes and very gentle pumping.

A sluggish lymphatic system can cause horrendous water retention that is certainly not eliminated by drinking water, as the experts say. The worst case is a condition called Lymphedema, which breast cancer patients sometimes end up with if they have had their lymph nodes removed.

To get the lymph moving, apart from the MLD massage, there are various devices that you can put on your legs and arms which pump the lymph to get it moving but they really do need to be used once a day. I have a pair of long boots that I bought from Cleo (the company who also supply face lift machines) that have a pumping action and ensure that the lymph is kept on the move. Remember that walking and general exercise will help as well.

Lymphatic problems can be helped with homeopathy and herbs, as listed below.

Other alternatives:

Homeopathy   Lymphomyosot from Elxirs.com

Herbs   Black walnut, burdock, cleavers, dandelion root

Lymph extract	As homeopathy or supplement
Other tips	Gentle Body brushing, Manual Lymphatic Drainage massage, exercise to keep lymph on the move, Exercise boots and arm sleeves
Detox	Lymphatic system detox
Louise Hay	A sluggish lymphatic system is a warning that the mind needs to be re-centred on the essentials of life, love and joy. So your affirmation will be "I am now totally centred in the love and joy of being alive. I flow with life"
Vitamins	All
Minerals	All

Gallbladder

The gallbladder is a small organ located just beneath the liver and it is connected to both the liver and the small intestine. The gallbladder stores and concentrates bile.

In response to cholecystokinin (a substance released into the blood when food is present in the stomach), the gallbladder contracts and bile is then pushed into the intestine. Digestion of fat occurs mainly in the small intestine, by pancreatic enzymes called lipases. The purpose of bile is to help the lipases to work, by emulsifying fat into smaller droplets to increase access for the enzymes Therefore, the gallbladder must break down the fat properly for general health. If it doesn't then you will have problems and could gain some weight.

Sometimes gallstones are formed and can cause problems both in and out of the gallbladder and I believe that the pain is absolutely terrible. You do have to be careful with some of the herbs because they may give you the pain of a trapped gallstone.

Other alternatives:

Homeopathy	Berberis vulgaris, Calcarea carbonica, Colocynthis
Herbs	Milk thistle, peppermint, turmeric
Gallbladder extract	Homeopathy or supplement
Detox	Detoxes are available for gallbladder
Vitamins	Vitamins A, D E and K
Minerals	All
Louise Hay	Gallbladder relates to bitterness therefore your affirmation will be "I joyously release of the past. Life is sweet and so am I".
Supplements	Be careful of the supplements you buy for the gallbladder. Sometimes they can bring on acute gallbladder pain similar to passing a stone.

Chapter 7:
BALANCE YOUR BRAIN CHEMISTRY FOR WEIGHT LOSS

Background

The science behind brain chemistry is very complex and there are masses of books that explain how it works much better than I ever could in a million years! If you would like to know more, these books are referenced at the end of the book.

My aim is to show you how important to your life and weight your brain chemistry is. Balanced brain chemistry improves your mood greatly, curbs your cravings and your appetite and helps you sleep better. And it will help you shed the weight efficiently and keep it off.

If you go to your doctor with depression or a weight problem, in the UK, they will never check your brain chemistry (or your vitamin/mineral levels come to that!). They may put you on anti-depressants and you may have heard that in some cases Prozac has been used for weight loss, but it is much simpler to balance your brain chemistry with either food or supplements or both to achieve better wellbeing and weight loss.

Then I started to investigate brain chemistry and it was like a light bulb being switched on in my head and it all made such perfect sense. Especially when you have been dieting for years, yo-yo dieting and starvation dieting, your brain chemistry gets depleted more and more over the years, making it difficult to lose weight or keep the weight off. This could explain why when somebody diets for the first time they get a good response but ten years down the line they are having trouble keeping the weight off or losing any more.

All that I have written here is about how your brain chemistry affects your appetite and how much you eat, which is scientific fact. However, from my personal experience I know that if your brain chemistry is not balanced you will not be able to lose any weight, even if you don't eat any more.

One of the causes of imbalanced brain chemistry is Seasonal Affected Disorder (commonly known as SAD) which affects a great number of people, usually between October and April, due mainly to lack of sunlight: sunlight helps in balancing brain chemistry. As a SAD sufferer from October to May, I would struggle with NOT EATING ANY MORE and yet I would put on at least 7 lbs over the winter. The problem then came when I wasn't exposed enough to the sun during the summer (I opened a beauty salon and never saw the light of day for four years!) and I didn't lose that 7lb. Over that four year period I put on two stone without eating another morsel. By this time my endocrine glands (see the chapter on how organs can affect our weight) were so low that even access to the sun couldn't raise them enough to relieve the SAD, so I started to put weight on during the summer as well, escalating this 'out of control' feeling from which I have suffered from for many years. As I have said many times in this book, I have a will of iron and I was determined not to put on any weight SO I WAS NOT OVEREATING like most of you who are reading this book.

Some of the information in this section may seem complicated but it is well worth sticking with it. If you would like more information there is a wealth of information on the internet.

What is brain chemistry?

Believe it or not but your brain chemistry can be one of the reasons that you put on weight and then can't lose it. People on low calorie diets miss meals and cut out protein in favour of lower calorie substitutes, such as a piece of toast. I was totally guilty of this, having lived for seven years on diet coke, a small tin diet tomato soup and a bag of low fat crisps because I craved salt – and I didn't lose an ounce of weight! Protein is even more important to people who are blood group O/Protein type in the eating plans that I recommend.

This is one reason why dieters gain weight as they don't get enough protein and calories to build and maintain muscle tissue, so the body starts burning muscle instead of using the fuel produced from carbohydrates.

As with every other therapy in this book you should consult a qualified nutritionalist/therapist who should be able to use tools like dowsing and muscle testing to get an accurate and personalised indication of the brain chemistry supplements needed.

Brain chemistry supplements can now be purchased from health food stores quite easily and chances are that if you are overweight/can't lose weight that you are lacking in at least two or maybe more. A chart is given later in this chapter outlining what problems you may have and what supplements will help solve that problem.

Food cravings

It might sound too good to be true but you can stop your food cravings almost instantly with just one supplement. Any absence in the brain chemistry needed sends powerful messages to quickly refuel your brain by eating refined carbohydrates.

Our biochemical response to food is triggered before we lift a fork. The sight, smell and anticipation of food stimulates the release of serotonin (a crucial part of your brain chemistry called a neurotransmitter) in the hypothalamus (a tiny part of the brain that oversees our eating and sleeping habits – more on the hypothalamus in the chapter on the endocrine system). Once we begin to eat, the serotonin levels continue to rise and then the hypothalamus sends out messages that your stomach is full and your craving has been satisfied. In other words you stop eating when your brain says that you are full and not your stomach.

So you can imagine the problems when your serotonin levels are insufficient. Other neurotransmitters also play a role in orchestrating appetite and food intake but serotonin appears to oversee the process. Research has shown that you can decrease food consumption by increasing serotonin activity in the brain and vice versa.

Once you correct your brain chemistry deficiencies, you will be free of food cravings, anxiety and you will be able to burn calories, lose fat and keep your muscle. You will also need to take various vitamins and minerals, which are outlined in the relevant chapter to help the supplements do their work.

Food for brain chemistry

A good way of getting your supply of brain chemistry requirements is with food, although if you are a serious dieter you are most probably so depleted of them that you will also need to take supplements for a while.

For the amino acids you need meat, milk, fish, eggs, poultry and cheese. These are called complete proteins and supply the essential nutrients in sufficient quantities.

Plant based proteins are usually missing one or more amino acids and are called incomplete proteins. But two or more plant based proteins can be combined together to create a complete protein, for example, pulses with whole grains, nuts or seeds combine to create complete protein.

When you are low on serotonin, you will crave carbohydrates so you need to recognise these signals and ensure that you have plenty of the right carbohydrates during the right time of the day.

What makes up brain chemistry?

Amino acids:
Amino acids are the 'building blocks' of the body. When protein is broken down by digestion the result is 22 known amino acids. Nine are essential (cannot be manufactured by the body) and the rest are non-essential (can be manufactured by the body with proper nutrition).

Neurotransmitters:
The four key mood chemicals (neurotransmitters) are made of amino acids and they also create and affect our moods:

Down in the dumps:
If you are high in dopamine and norepinephrine (neurotransmitters) you are good, happy and alert.
If you are low in dopamine and norepinephrine you are at your lowest ebb possible and will be definitely down in the dumps

Anxiety and Stress:
If you are high in GABA (a neurotransmitter) you're relaxed and stress-free – hurrah!
If you are low in GABA you'll be overwhelmed and twitchy

Oversensitive Feelings:
If you are high in endorphins you're so happy and high
If you are low in endorphins you will be tearful and over sensitive

Depression:

> If you are high in Serotonin you're positive, confident, flexible and easy-going
>
> If you are low in Serotonin you'll tend to become negative, obsessive, worried, irritable and can't sleep

If we have enough of the above four neurotransmitters we are stable and happy. However, serial dieting or an imbalance can affect quite considerably how we feel. We can crave foods such as sweets or carbohydrates to give us a buzz and an imbalance can cause you to crave alcohol and drugs and become addictive.

Some examples of how they can help:

L'glutamine can reach a starving brain within minutes and puts a stop to cravings – hurrah!

L-tyrosine produces thyroid and adrenaline – the thyroid controlling the metabolism and therefore essential for weight loss and maintenance

Serotonin stops cravings and makes us feel self confident and happy

Examples of how deficiencies in neurotransmitters and amino acids manifest themselves

Deficiency symptoms	Addictive substances used	What amino acids/neurotransmitters to take	Positive outcome
Craving for sugar, starch or alcohol Moodiness from low blood sugar Overeating Weight gain	Sweets Starches Alcohol	L-glutamine	Stable blood sugars, calm, alert brain function Weight loss
Depression Lack of energy Lack of drive Lack of focus/ concentration Attention deficit disorder	Sweets Starch Chocolate Aspartame Alcohol Marijuana and other	L-tyrosine L-phenylalanine	Happiness Energy Mental focus

Increased appetite Weight gain	drugs Caffeine Cigarettes		Drive Weight loss
Stressed and burned out Unable to relax/ loosen up Still and tense muscles Weight gain	Sweets Starch Cigarettes Marijuana Valium Alcohol	GABA	Calmness Relaxation
Very sensitive to emotional or physical pain Cry easily Crave comfort, reward or numbing treats Addicted to certain foods or drugs	Sweets/chocol ate Carbs Alcohol Marijuana and other drugs Cigarettes	DL-phenylalanine D-phenylalanine	Happiness Physical pain relief Pleasure Reward Loving feelings
Negativity Depression Worry/ anxiety, Low self-esteem, Obsessive thoughts/behavi our Seasonal Affect Disorder (SAD) Thyroid problems PMS Weight gain Overeating Brain fog Irritability/ rage Heat intolerance Panic, phobias Afternoon or evening cravings	Sweets Starch Chocolate Alcohol Marijuana Ecstasy Cigarettes	L-tryptophan 5-HTP converts into Serotonin Melatonin for sleep at bedtimes	Feel like a million dollars Emotional stability Self confidence Weight loss Good sleep (made from serotonin)

Fibromyalgia, TMJ Night-owl, hard to get to sleep Insomnia, disturbed sleep Suicidal thoughts Jet lag			

Taking amino acid supplements

Amino acid supplements should be taken out of the capsule and placed under the tongue. They should not be taken with food but the meal following should contain good protein.

Start by taking one amino acid supplement per day to be sure of the effects before you start the next one. It would be a good idea to record what you do in your journal. Follow the instructions carefully as they may be absorbed better if they are taken at a certain time of day.

Amino acid supplements are only needed temporarily and should be tapered off when you are feeling better but you should stay on them for a minimum of three months to give you chance to feel the benefits. You may have to take L-tryptophan or 5-HTP in the winter months to counteract SAD.

It would be preferable to cut out alcohol and any other stimulants altogether. If you follow the guidelines in this book for supplements you will find that your craving for alcohol will diminish.

Using amino acid contraindications
If you suffer with the following, please consult a doctor before taking any supplements:
- High blood pressure
- Low blood pressure
- Migraine headaches
- Severe, manic depression or any other mental illness
- If you have any severe illness of any organ or cancer
- If you are taking any medication for mood problems

- If you are pregnant or nursing
- If you are taking St Johns wort

A supplement should contain the amino acids that you require including the nine essential ones that are needed.

Always inform your doctor if you are taking any medication including homeopathy or herbs. This is very important because taking lots of tablets can cause interactions that might make you ill. If you feel ill at anytime immediately come off any non-doctor prescribed medication.

The nine essential amino acids are:

Lysine
Lysine ensures the adequate absorption of calcium; helps form collagen (which makes up bone cartilage and connective tissues – also stops you aging!); aids in the production of antibodies, hormones & enzymes. Recent studies have shown that Lysine may be effective against herpes by improving the balance of nutrients that reduce viral growth. A deficiency may result in tiredness, inability to concentrate, irritability, bloodshot eyes, retarded growth, hair loss, anemia and reproductive problems.

Phenylalanine
(also referred to as L-phenylalanine, D-phenlylalanine (DPA) and DL-phenlylalanine (DLPA))

This is used by the brain to produce Norepinephrine, a chemical that transmits signals between nerve cells and the brain; keeps you awake & alert; reduces hunger pains; functions as an antidepressant and helps improve memory.

Leucine & Threonine
This is an important constituent of collagen, Elastin, and enamel protein; helps prevents fat build-up in the liver; helps the digestive and intestinal tracts function more smoothly; assists metabolism and assimilation.

New research shows that animals injected with leucine ate 20% less food the following day and only gained a third of the weight of their peers after a 24-hour fast. Leucine acts on the enzyme mTOR which is highly active in the hypothalamus which regulates the appetite. So this amino acid could be more beneficial for weight loss than previously thought.

Isoleucine
This provides ingredients for the manufacturing of other essential biochemical components in the body, some of which are utilised for the production of energy, stimulants to the upper brain and helping you to be more alert.

Tryptophan (precursor of Serotonin – Supplement referred to as 5-HTP)
A natural relaxant, helps alleviate insomnia by inducing normal sleep; reduces anxiety & depression; helps in the treatment of migraine headaches; helps the immune system; helps reduce the risk of artery & heart spasms; works with Lysine in reducing cholesterol levels.

Methionine
Methionine is a principle supplier of sulphur which prevents disorders of the hair, skin and nails; helps lower cholesterol levels by increasing the liver's production of lecithin; reduces liver fat and protects the kidneys; a natural chelating agent for heavy metals; regulates the formation of ammonia and creates ammonia-free urine which reduces bladder irritation; influences hair follicles and promotes hair growth.

Histidine
Is found abundantly in hemoglobin; has been used in the treatment of rheumatoid arthritis, allergic diseases, ulcers & anemia. A deficiency can cause poor hearing.

Valine
Promotes mental vigor, muscle coordination and calm emotions.

Arginine
Is considered to be essential in infants and helps to release the fat burning hormone glucagons into your blood and helps circulation.

Also essential for losing weight:

L-tyrosine
transmits nerve impulses to the brain; helps overcome depression; Improves memory; increases mental alertness; promotes the healthy functioning of the thyroid, adrenal and pituitary glands

L-Carnosine

This is a natural body product consisting of the amino acids Beta-alanine and L-histidine chemically bound together. Apart from helping collagen, regenerating cells, a zinc and copper regulator, a super antioxidant it also helps to flush toxins from the body. Now famed as an anti-ager and weight loss supplement as well.

This is being hailed as the new anti-ageing way to go and there are also rumours that it can banish cellulite. I don't know about that but I am definitely going to check it out and could be buying it in bulk!

L-glutamine

Is considered to be nature's 'brain food' by improving mental capacities; helps speed the healing of ulcers; gives a 'lift' from fatigue; helps control alcoholism, schizophrenia and the craving for sugar

L-Carnitine

This is involved in the metabolism of food into energy. It also contributes to the production of a neurotransmitter which is required for mental function. L-Carnitine contributes to the production of the brain neurotransmitter Acetylcholine so may increase mental function. Assists in the metabolism of food into energy, and enhances Glucose uptake in type II diabetes. This amino acid helps to shift long fatty acids to be burnt by the body - an aid to fat burning. If you don't have this and chromium the nutrients won't get into your cells. Also good for weight loss.

5-HTP

This is about 5 to 10 times more powerful than tryptophan. However it is possible to increase the serotonin which can produce side effects. Start on a low dose (25 to 50 milligrams) and increase the dose slowly every 3 to 5 days to a maximum of 200 milligrams.

You can feel the benefit of 5-HTP within an hour but you must give it a fair chance. I can't remember the number of people who have started to take supplements and if they don't feel like a 25 year old in a week they stop taking them!

Melatonin

Melatonin is the natural sleeping pill. In the afternoon and the evening, serotonin is converted into melatonin and therefore you need extra supplies. As serotonin levels begin to decline, you become low in serotonin and then crave carbohydrates which will give you that temporary lift. If 5-HTP or St John's Wort do not level out your sleeping problems you may need to take 0.5 to 3 mgs of melatonin. Melatonin is now used widely as a cure for jet lag. Use of light boxes after midday and the screens of mobile gadgets can negatively affect your melatonin levels and you will not be able to sleep.

Vitamin B6
Vitamin B6 helps the body convert 5-HTP into serotonin in the brain so it would be helpful to take a B complex as you need all the B vitamins to work in harmony.

Herbs and Homeopathy

The best herb and homeopathy remedy to raise serotonin levels is St John's Wort. A mass of research has been published about the effectiveness about this herb, especially for SAD sufferers. I would highly recommend it.

Contra-indications: Do not take St John Wort if you are on the contraceptive pill as it negates the effectiveness and you could find yourself pregnant! It also increases your sensitivity to light so beware if you are sunbathing or on holiday (you shouldn't need to take it if you are in sunny country as the sunlight has the same effect on your brain chemistry). I speak from experience here because I burnt a rather nasty hole in my leg on holiday in Mauritius when taking St John's Wort and it took a while to heal.

Light box

The best way I have found of raising my serotonin levels is to be in sunlight for as long as possible – which is virtually impossible in the English summer! However, you can now buy a light box which you can use (but do not look into it) and I have just purchased a light alarm clock so that I am woken up to sunrise and I go to sleep to sunset, which is another way to balance the Serotonin levels.

Use the light box during the first half of the day as you will confuse your body if you use it later and you will not be able to sleep.

Exercise

Exercise helps raise serotonin levels and improves your mood so ensure that you include some form of exercise every day – preferably outside like a walk at lunchtime

Conclusion

When all your amino acids and neurotransmitters are balanced you are feeling happy and on the way to losing your fat and water retention but keeping your muscle tissue.

They also have many other functions which are covered at length on sites on the internet which is where I would suggest you look if you want to know more, because in this book I am only interested in helping weight loss.

Chapter 8:
ALLERGIES AND INTOLERANCES

Information about allergies and intolerances is very important for losing weight and then maintaining that weight loss. This is because they can add weight and water as part of their reaction and it will stay firmly as water or fat until the allergy or intolerance is eliminated. Luckily, there are now many ways of identifying allergies and intolerances and then you have a choice. You either investigate how to heal it or leave it out of your diet (if it is food – nothing much I can advise for wasp stings except keep away from wasps!).

Allergies and intolerances are rising to almost epidemic proportions, especially in children. A lot of research on this seems to point to vaccines given to babies and young children and then to other medicines, such as antibiotics and steroids which break down the immune system. This in turn makes us unable to cope with food and substances like we did years ago. We are full of toxins and poisons from our everyday lives. Our gut flora is compromised and this has been proven to affect the immune system as well. There can also be an emotional aspect. For example, asthma can be related to not wanting to breathe or holding onto your breath to get attention or to avoid something you don't want to do.

I was told that when I was young that the milk powder I was given set up an allergy which multiplied my fat cells. Remember, protein powders can contain dairy product so if you have a problem with dairy always check their contents before taking.

What is the difference between an allergy and an intolerance?

An **allergy** is an abnormal immune system response to the introduction of a food or another substance (such as cat hair) to the body. A reaction can occur within minutes or a few hours after the food or substance is ingested. An **intolerance** is an adverse reaction to a food or substance that does not involve the immune system. Reactions can be immediate or delayed up to twenty hours after a food or the substance is ingested.

Intolerances are more common than realised – for example two in four people will have some sort of sensitivity to dairy products or wheat.

How to diagnose an allergy or intolerance

These are the general ways that they are diagnosed:
- Blood test from a 3rd party – these are pretty accurate but are very expensive
- Prick test – where they put food and substance particles on your skin to see your reactions – can be limited and not cover a wide enough area
- Dowsing with a crystal pendulum – this is a wonderful way of finding out whether something suits you or not
- Muscle testing (also called Kinesiology) – Muscle testing is normally carried out while the patient is holding a phial with the substance in it. The muscle is moved slightly to see if it is strong or weak. A weak muscle denotes an allergy or intolerance. I have boxes and boxes of phials of a vast array of foods and substances to which people can be allergic/intolerant, so this is another very thorough way of identifying what is causing the problem

Common symptoms

The symptoms relating to intolerances and allergies are not limited to those shown below but the list does cover the most important ones relating to weight and water gain.
- Bloating & weight gain
- Water retention and oedema
- Skin rashes and serious problems such as eczema and psoriasis
- Digestive problems, IBS and Crohn's disease
- Sneezing & hay fever
- Depression and headaches
- Phlegm and sinus problems
- Joint and bone pain
- Asthma & other breathing problems

Common allergies

Obviously you can be allergic to any substance but these are the most common ones:
- Nuts, especially peanuts

- Stings (wasp and bee)
- Substances such as diesel, fuel and carpet cleaner
- Pet hair
- Gluten
- Dairy
- Yeast & wheat
- Face creams
- Hair dyes
- Grass, grass seed and blossom (especially rape seed)

Common intolerances

As mentioned before, you can be intolerant to any substance but these are the most common ones:

- Milk and dairy products
- Eggs
- Fruit & vegetables
- Monosodium glutamate
- Aspartame
- Colours, preservatives and additives
- Pet hair
- Substances like fuel, diesel and carpet cleaner
- Air fresheners
- Washing powders and conditioners
- Yeast & wheat

Histamine

Histamine is a chemical which occurs naturally in certain foods. It is also one of the chemicals that is released in the body as part of an allergic reaction, causing the typical itching, sneezing, wheezing and swelling allergy symptoms. Recently it has been discovered that you can be intolerant to your own histamine and not many doctors know about it. In a recent Daily Mail article a young lady had chronic eczema and was always tired and bloated. She suffered for many years until she met a doctor that had just heard of histamine intolerance. Histamine enters the body through various types of food, such as red wine and beer, cheese, yeast, chocolate, cured meats, shellfish and most fish. The young lady eventually cured herself by cutting out these foods and cooking only fresh meals. This would be a good one to mention to your practitioner.

Eliminating allergies and intolerances

Luckily there is now a wealth of available therapies and techniques that will help you eliminate allergies and intolerances – although allergies may prove to be more stubborn than intolerances to shift.

However, you will also have to test yourself on a regular basis if you have serious life threatening allergies like peanuts, wasp stings and any others that affect you really badly. I would never suggest that you start eating peanuts on a regular basis even though your allergy will be better – better safe than sorry. You will also need to supplement your diet with vitamins, minerals, probiotics (kefir) and food enzymes.

Please also remember that the start of the allergy/intolerance may have resulted at the same time as an emotional incident in your life, so when using EFT™, try and identify an emotional cause as well as a physical one.

For example, you could have an intolerance to milk that started when you were six. When you look at this further you might realise that you were drinking milk the day you were told that your grandfather had died. The shock and trauma of this news set off a future intolerance to milk.

Recommended by the medical profession
Withdraw from lifestyle of food or substances.

Tested and recommended by myself
All the techniques I talk about here are explained in more detail throughout this book. Emotional Freedom Technique (EFT™) in my mind is the most useful as it eliminates the emotional and the physical problems.

EFT™:
Even though I am allergic/intolerant to '......', I deeply and utterly love and accept myself and I chose for my body to accept '............'

Homeopathy
There are various homeopathy remedies that you can take for hay fever, pet hair and other substances. I haven't tried these but I know that homeopaths have great results with them. Either contact a trained homeopath or Helios Pharmacy, who will recommend what type of remedy and the dose for you (see Appendix V).

The slow poisoning of America by **Michelle and John Erb**
Please read this book as it is absolutely fascinating. It talks about all the additives, colours and preservatives in our food and how they are making us ill with digestive and skin problems, plus weight and water gain. Michelle and John Erb's main concerns are that they are all addictive and that the food companies are adding them to our food so that we will eat more. This has got to stop and you can start now by choosing a healthy fresh diet and chose not to buy pre-packaged and processed foods.

Other concerns are MSG and Aspartame which are to be found in a vast number of foods and drinks we buy, even those that are not essentially sweet products. Aspartame contained in a sweetener stopped my kidneys working in just a couple of months – to me that shows how dangerous they are – especially when it is being ingested by all our children. .

MSG
When scientists inject new-born rats or mice with monosodium glutamate (MSC) they become obese. Rats and mice are not naturally obese but MSG triples the amount of insulin. This in turn makes the rats/mice obese and could it do it to humans as well. Not only is it addictive, it also sends your insulin wild so that you need more food – it really is a vicious circle!

MSG is mainly known for being added to Chinese cuisine. Why do they add it and in such large quantities? Because MSG is addictive and it will make you eat more eat more. That could be why a couple of hours after a Chinese meal you feel hungry again.

Be warned that Hydrolysed Vegetable Protein is another name for MSG.

Not only can MSG make you eat more but you can have an intolerance to it which causes all sorts of side effects such as bloating, digestive problems and skin rashes.

My experience with MSG is quite frightening as it slows down all my bodily functions, I feel ill and lethargic and don't move my bowels for two days. It also seems to affect my kidneys and bladder and stops me passing water. I find, too, that I become incredibly hungry, which backs up the research.

As with many of the subjects, I have not got the space to discuss all aspects so do your research on the internet to find out the full details.

MSG really is the most dreadful stuff and should be banned from all products NOW!

Aspartame

This is used as a sweetener in nearly everything from spreads to low calorie drinks. According to my research it accounts for approximately 70% of ALL complaints to the FDA and is responsible for a wide variety of problems from headaches to Parkinson's or MS. Aspartame is sold under various well-known brand names. The most worrying thing is that it breaks down within twenty minutes at room temperature into several primary toxic and dangerous ingredients – and we are feeding this to our children, too.

As I am writing this it has just dawned on me that since I have gone back to sugar I don't have any headaches. When I was taking a major brand of sweetener, it stopped my kidneys working properly. This was extremely frightening and even now I have to support my kidneys with herbs at all times and if I inadvertently eat or drink something with aspartame in it, I immediately get pain in my kidney area.

Aspartame also makes you very hungry, so beware. Don't swap the diet drinks for the full sugar ones as they are so calorific and will also make you hungry. Cut out fizzy drinks altogether and drink water and small amount of good quality fruit juice. Also I just read an article which says that drinking fizzy drinks gives women brittle bones – another reason for throwing them out of your diet.

Alternative to all sweeteners and sugar is Stevia (a South America herb) and Xylitol (extracted from plant materials) – they have been proven to be very safe and can be used in cooking as well as drinks. Stevia also balances your sugar levels (insulin) as well, so it kills two birds with one stone. Xylitol is also good for your teeth and has been added to chewing gum.

Please read *Sweet Deception* by Joseph Mercola which is full of the most amazing facts about how all the sweeteners were discovered and, believe me, it's frightening.

Fluoride

Fluoride has been added to our tap water for years and is causing many problems. It can cause wheezing and skin complaints and, more seriously, can lower IQ and cause depression. It absolutely degrades the thyroid and slows down the metabolism. Unfortunately most filters don't take out fluoride so you may need to drink bottled water. Please ensure that the water is in a glass bottle so you are not consuming too much plastic.

Colours, preservatives and other additives

From looking at the two sections above you can see that eating or drinking anything with colours, preservatives and additives is going to be bad for you. At best they may make you itch or swell but if you have an intolerance to them the effects can be much worse. Be extra careful of fizzy drinks that are coloured. If you absolutely have to drink a fizzy drink make sure it is clear rather than coloured.

Mixed intolerances

This is a very interesting subject and one that is not picked up with the blood or the prick tests, as you are not allergic/intolerant to the items on their own. For example, you eat cheese and bread separately and you are absolutely fine. However, when you eat a cheese sandwich you fall asleep immediately. It means that combining those two foods together makes you intolerant to them. This can happen with lots of combinations of food types.

That's what happens with cola. Very often children don't show intolerance to each ingredient of cola when you are doing muscle testing, for example. But when the ingredients are combined, you get a resounding big 'no'!

Keep a journal

Even if you eliminate your allergies/food intolerances it is still a good idea to keep them out of your diet for a couple of months and then re-introduce them slowly. Keep a food diary of what you are eating, how it affects you and what you do about it. This is very important to keep yourself in tip top shape. If you are following the correct eating plan for you and eliminate your intolerances you should find that you will have no excess water retention or digestive problems and should start to lose weight.

Chapter 9:
HOW HORMONES AFFECT YOUR WEIGHT

Background

Hormones are where men gain a distinct advantage over us women! PMS and the menopause with its weight gain, water retention, mood swings and cravings means that not only can women not lose weight on certain weeks of their cycle but sometimes actually put on weight, which then becomes very difficult to lose. Men have the ability to lose weight all month and also because of their hormones they distribute fat differently and don't have cellulite – next time I am definitely coming back as a man!

My horrific experience

I would most probably say that my hormones have caused me more trouble than all of my other problems put together. It was when I start puberty at a very early age that I put on a tremendous amount of weight and from then on I could never lose it. Also at that time I started the headaches, migraines, PMS and horrendous water retention just for good measure!

My hormonal water retention and symptoms lasted for three weeks per month. My boobs were so sore that I could scream. My fingers and ankles filled up with so much water they would go bright red and throb until I wanted to cut them off. My stomach would swell until I looked pregnant and it was rock hard.

I then had cravings, so it was a constant battle, not just of not eating but also craving carbohydrates and sweets so much I didn't know what to do with myself. Then there was the depression and bad temper that got worse as the month progressed.

I had never sweated, due to my thyroid problem but then I hit the menopause and started to sweat during both the night and the day, which I found particularly revolting. The water retention then got even worse, if that was possible, so much so that the only shoes I could wear were black casual sandals. The sandals looked absolutely ridiculous, especially when I was walking through the rain in open sandals and, because I am a girl that loves shoes, it broke my heart to look at fifty pairs of beautiful coloured shoes I couldn't wear that were sitting there in my bedroom.

The minute my period finished, the symptoms would start again and get worse as the month progressed. I tried Dong Quai and put on a stone in one month. I tried Black Cohosh and got the most terrible headaches. Then, of course, came the time when I couldn't take any medication at all, not even the vitamins that are essential for the menstrual cycle and so the symptoms ran riot.

How to stop the misery of the monthly cycle

There is a whole lot of help available now on balancing hormones but it is essential that it is done on an individual basis for you with your diagnostic tools. One herb may work for one but not for another so your testing must be pretty accurate. You may have to try a couple of herbs or remedies before you get one that suits you perfectly.

Go to Sandra Cabot's website at http://www.weightcontroldoctor.com and see how she tests hormonal levels in her clinics with saliva tests – I wish she had a clinic in England! I have never been offered to have my hormones tested by saliva or any other method.

Why do hormones give us so much grief?

The main female hormones that we have change in relationship during the month but the main problems arise when they get out of balance, especially when you become oestrogen dependant. That means that you have too much oestrogen in your body. This can be caused by many factors, including the pill and HRT, other medication, poor diet and stress. Sometimes it means that the endocrine organs that produce your hormones can be out of balance and they will need to be addressed first.

Oestrogen is mainly responsible for many of the PMS symptoms, bloating, cravings, weight and water gain and crying., Progesterone, on the other hand, is good for the metabolism so if you have too low a level your system is not burning food efficiently.

In the UK the doctors do not test your homes before they put you on the pill or HRT so they have no idea whether the medication will give you other problems! Do not be frightened to keep going back until you find the mediation that suits you.

Another hormone that can cause us ladies problems is testosterone, believe it or not. This can cause low libido and other side effects and is often overlooked, especially if there is a hormonal imbalance after childbirth. So ask your doctor to be tested for this hormone as well. Testosterone is not just a male hormone.

The endocrine system and hormones

During the chapter on the endocrine system I describe how the organs and all the hormones they produce are intertwined and finely tuned – it's really quite amazing that our bodies work at all. When your hormones are imbalanced sometimes you need to look higher up the chain and ask other questions such as is it my:

- Thyroid
- Hypothalamus
- Pituitary
- Pineal, or
- Adrenals

that is causing these problems (or a combination, as they are closely linked)? Then you have to act accordingly. Stored fat can also produce oestrogen and that can add to the problem as well. You can take supplements but the symptoms never go away because you have to get the other organ(s) working correctly. That in turn will balance the hormones and you will generally feel much better.

Vitamins & minerals

Calcium, zinc, magnesium and B vitamins are all essential to aid the monthly cycle and menopausal symptoms. There are various supplements that combine all of these together and I would recommend that you take them every day. Most of us are short of these vitamins because we are not eating so much protein (especially red meat) and are eating more junk food. You will notice the difference immediately. Zinc is especially good for raising the libido which normally goes out of the window when you have horrendous PMS symptoms!

Evening primrose oil or star oil is also essential for PMS as it gives you the fatty acid that you need. You will most probably find that you will need to take this and omega-3 oils, especially at the beginning.

Watch your iron levels as well because PMS and menopausal symptoms can cause anaemia, as does low thyroid function. Taking iron tablets may cause constipation so you may want to look at eating iron rich food or take a particular homeopathic remedy called cell salts.

There are various food alternatives in the chapter on vitamins and minerals but I do feel that certainly to begin with you need to have additional help in the form of supplements.

Herbs and homeopathy

When looking for any remedy you need one that will balance your hormones and not simply fill you full of oestrogen as do the pill and HRT. This is where your diagnostic tools will come in very handy. These herbs and homeopathic remedies are all available in tablet form so you don't have to boil up any leaves as was done in the past!

Blue cohosh:
Good for PMS symptoms and it doesn't seem to have the contrain-dications that Black cohosh has: works on relieving the pain in the legs caused by water retention.

Sarsaprilla:
Saponins and plant steroids found in sarsaparilla can be synthesised into human steroids, such as oestrogen and testosterone, which will help PMS symptoms.

Dong quai:
Don quai is supposed to balance hormones but I found that it pumped extra oestrogen into the body. I suffered from water retention after taking this product and put on a stone in a month, so I don't particularly recommend it, but it might suit you.

Black cohosh:
Black cohosh has been shown to help with menopausal symptoms, such as hot flushes, irritability and balancing oestrogen levels.

You must only stay on this remedy for a maximum of six months. It can cause severe headaches and in extreme cases can cause a heart attack.

In my experience this herb didn't balance my levels but gave me headaches and I did swell up with water, although not as much as I did with dong quai. However, this herb is very successful for many people.

Wild and Mexican yam:
Supposed to contain progesterone which is to balance women with oestrogen dominance (ie too much oestrogen). There are various articles on the internet which questions the substance and even say that it actually contain oestrogen as well as progesterone, so just be careful.

Maca: *This is the one that I take and highly recommend*
This is a South American herb and it is brilliant because it gets the pituitary and thyroid to work and to produce the correct hormones. It is mainly used for menopausal symptoms (this is the remedy that I use for my menopausal symptoms. It also brings back the libido!). Maca is excellent for the relief of the following menopausal problems:
• Night sweats / hot flushes
• Fatigue
• Memory lapse / mood swings
• Correct oestrogen dominance
• Osteoporosis

The American doctor, Gabriel Cousens, prefers Maca to hormone replacement therapy (HRT). He states: "Maca is a balanced answer to the effects of an ageing endocrine system. HRT declines the capacity of the endocrine glands to produce hormones; this fosters the ageing of the body".

Agnus Castus:*
The effect it has on female hormones is largely a balancing effect. This is a herb that I have used with success and would highly recommend.

Agnus Castus can improve the following PMS symptoms:
• Headaches and migraines
• Breast tenderness
• Fatigue
• Bloating
• Anxiety and other similar psychological symptoms

- Irregular cycle
- Agnus Castus can improve:
- Night sweats / hot flushes (flashes)
- Fatigue

Other herbs

There are other herbs, such as red clover and raspberry leaf but I think the main ones are listed above – certainly the ones I would recommend. Raspberry leaf comes into its own for an easy labour – just remember that if you are pregnant!

Water tablets

It is recommended that you may take some form of herbal diuretic to relieve the monthly water retention. If you are on a herb or homeopathic remedy it should also help to sort out your water retention. If these don't work you need to change the remedy you are taking.

Lachesis

This is a highly recommended homeopathic remedy that is given for all sorts of hormonal complaints (plus fear of snakes as it comes from snake venom!). Highly recommended for PMS and menopause systems

Fatty Acids

Taking a supplement of evening primrose oil, starflower oil and/or fish oil will help stop PMS symptoms and boost the metabolism in the menopause. These oils are a must in everybody's diet.

Soya

Soya has been hailed as some form of miracle for PMS and menopause systems and some people swear by it, so you must try it to see if it is good for you.

However, my experience of soya hasn't been good and I list the reasons below:

- Many people have an intolerance/allergy to Soya (I have an intolerance).
- It lowers the thyroid function which you don't want even if you have a brilliant thyroid, let alone if it doesn't work properly!
- It decreases your DHEA level, as well as other hormones in menstruating women
- It can increase breast cancer

- It is difficult to digest
- It can be genetically modified which I wouldn't touch with a barge pole!

I wouldn't recommend eating soya as part of your hormonal plan and only eat it in very small amounts for health reasons. If soya helps you then just make sure you do not have an intolerance to it.

A new discovery

Professor Millar, director of the Human Reproductive Sciences Unit at the Medical Research Council in Edinburgh has found, by testing on animals, that Type 2 Gonadotropin-releasing hormone increased libido (the imagination boggles at how they test this!) and aided weight loss. This seems to be achieved by cutting appetite by a third. Sounds like the answer to most men's prayer – a slim women who is randy! However, the weight loss does seem to be achieved by cutting appetite rather than curing the hormonal imbalance. Watch this space to see if it comes out on the market.

Natural oestrogen and progesterone creams

If you don't want to go down the herbal or homeopathic route, for hormones it is better to use a cream on certain weeks of the month, rather than take a pill every day or use a patch. Always go for the natural option and not the synthetic option.

As mentioned earlier in this chapter I would suggest that you read the books *What doctors don't tell you about the menopause* and *PMS*. They are full of interesting facts and advise on what type of creams to buy and why not to take HRT.

Supplements can be given for the following hormones from your therapist. Natural hormones are more preferable to synthetic hormones. Natural progesterone is available in chemists and natural oestrogen and testosterone would have to be specially ordered. Please note that progesterone increases metabolism – good for people with low thyroids.

There are three types of naturally occurring oestrogen: oestradiol, oestriol and oestrone and these three can be blended together. Creams build up very quickly so do get regular testing if you use either oestrogen or progesterone cream.

- Progesterone
- Oestrogen
- Testosterone
- Oestriol
- Oestradiol

HRT

In my opinion, HRT pumps the body full of oestrogen that it doesn't need. Most HRT is either totally oestrogen or oestrogen dependant and this is the state that you are trying to avoid. Although doctors deny this, the menopause and HRT can cause weight gain that is virtually impossible to get rid of. When I had my beauty salon, I met many menopausal ladies that suffered with their weight and were given no support by their GP.

There have been many scares recently in various reports saying that HRT can cause breast cancer and other problems, that it isn't good for bone density and it has been proven to increase the risk of asthma in older women, which is why asthma is now on the increase in older women. There is a lot of research on the internet which I suggest you read. However, if you feel that you need to take HRT please follow your doctor's instructions and if you decided to come off it, reduce your dose slowly and look for other alternatives.

The contraceptive pill

Funnily enough, the pill really suited me because, as my hormones were low, the pill increased my oestrogen level to over 98% which is the cut off point for most of my PMS symptoms. I lost my water retention, consequently lost weight and felt marvellous. However, for most women it pumps you full of oestrogen, which you don't need, and has many of side effects, including weight gain and over eating.

It is a good idea to find some other form of contraception that isn't so evasive and if you are taking the pill for period problems, perhaps you should investigate alternatives.

What do I mean by 98%?

As you know, I use a pendulum to dowse and during the seventeen year period of training, I could measure at what level my body got better and the symptoms elevated. I knew that if my oestrogen level got over 98% that the water retention would become virtually non-existent, the sore boobs would disappear totally and then the nearer to a 100% I got all the other symptoms would go as well. However, when you start to go over 100% of oestrogen, the symptoms begin to appear again, with massive water retention and not being able to lose weight being the main problems.

The importance of balance and proper testing

The balance between the hormones is absolutely vital. Taking any form of medication or alternative can affect the balance and it may cure one symptom only to be met with another one.

There are other hormones to be balanced as well, including testosterone and DHEA. Especially when women approach the menopause, the adrenals are then responsible for producing oestrogen and progesterone and if they are not in good condition (ie exhausted or stressed), they will also cause an imbalance. Because of lifestyles the adrenals are becoming exhausted. Also if you have a low thyroid you use your adrenals for energy and therefore this causes exhaustion as well.

Testing

Doctor blood test:
These are very difficult to get in the UK and sometimes the results are not accurate as they can record inactive as well as active hormones. You can pay for them to be done privately but this can be very expensive.

Saliva testing:
I would recommend that at some time you have a saliva test to check your hormones.

Muscle testing/dowsing:
Go to an experienced therapist who can accurate define what levels and balance your hormones are at. They can then test for the relevant alternatives that you need

Vega machine (or equivalent testing machine):
These use a pointer that is attached to the meridian line (similar to those used in acupuncture) which gives accurate readings of the status of your organs, hormones and vitamin levels – they are brilliant and I would highly recommend them. These are normally used by homeopaths to check levels and then test the remedies they recommend.

Eating for hormones

In my case, what I ate didn't make the slightest difference because my hormone level was so low and unbalanced that I needed more help. However, if your levels are only slightly imbalanced it is worth a try.

You also will know about the cravings and how you can eat a chocolate bar and not realise you have eaten it – we have all done it at some time to satisfy the urge. You will be craving foods like fats, sugars, artificial sweeteners, flour, caffeine and chocolate.

If you take the amino acid and mineral and vitamin supplements you will find that your cravings virtually disappear.
- L-glutamine stops the craving for sweets, starches and alcohol
- 5-HTP improves your mood
- St John's Wort raises serotonin levels
- GABA relaxes your muscles like a natural valium and increases pain relief
- D-phenylalanine will increase pain relief
- L-tyrosine will help you with caffeine cravings
- Chromium also stops the cravings and stops you feeling hungry

Refer to the chapter on brain chemistry to see which ones you will need to fit your symptoms.

Eat a healthy diet with protein, fresh fruit and vegetables and whole grains. This should correspond to the eating plan that you have decided to adopt.

Remember that eating a diet too high in carbohydrate will keep you hormonally imbalanced. Excess dieting or unhealthy eating will also cause you problems, so eat three balanced meals a day.

If taking the supplements, amino acids and eating sensibly doesn't cure all your craving (or other symptoms for that matter) you can use EFT™ with wonderful results.

Keep a log

It is really important to keep a monthly log and record how you feel emotionally and physically, and the reactions you may be having with your medication. Do you feel better, are there improvements or do you feel worse? You then adjust your medication accordingly, have another saliva test or visit your therapist for accurate diagnosis. If you don't keep a log you will not be able to map your progress.

If your hormones are too high, stop eating any food or taking any supplements or herbs that might be encouraging excess (hormonal creams are particularly suspect).
* Increase the amount of vitamin C for a few months
* Eat plenty of fibre foods
* Try Biocare's Phosphatidal Serine Precursor or Phos Serine Complex by Allergy Research Group which can bring down excessive cortisol levels.

Sunlight

As I explained in my introduction, when I had access to over three hours of sunlight a day, my PMS symptoms disappeared immediately and I felt like a million dollars. I didn't get the same affect with a light box, although there was some improvement.

This shows that the endocrine system is boosted considerably by the sun. Therefore try to spend as much time in the sun as you possibly can, some of that time without protection (early morning and late evening)

Exercise

Exercise will raise the serotonin levels (only temporarily though) so try to include moderate exercise all through your cycle, even though you most probably will not feel like it.

Relaxation

Take up relaxation tapes, meditation and perhaps Yoga as the less stressed you are, the better your hormones will work.

Body types

When you look around, you will see that everybody is made differently. Some people have a tiny top and a big bottom half, some people are straight up and down, some curvy etc (and we are not usually the one we want to be!).

Most of these body types relate to our hormones and there is more information about body types in Chapter 5. However, you normally find that the people with a small top and bigger bottom are oestrogen dependant and that is why they are distributing fat on their bottom.

This would explain why we can't spot reduce or lose weight or fat in certain areas. Also, during the menopause you put more fat on the tummy, even if you have had no excess weight problem all your life.

We have all been on diets where you lose all the weight off your face, but none goes from your legs or your bottom. Hopefully by balancing your hormones and eating for your body type/metabolic type and doing the right exercise you will be able to see more of a balance in your body.

Cellulite

In my opinion cellulite is caused mainly by hormones and then by toxins and trapped water. Once again, when you have balanced your hormones, eating correctly and drinking water (plus body brushing and the various cellulite creams that are on the market) you should see a marked improvement.

Clay body wraps are good for cellulite (but don't have them when you have PMT otherwise you won't lose the trapped water).

You most probably will also need to do a cleanse and detox every now and again to make sure that you are healthy. Cut down on alcohol and caffeine.

Other therapies

I have tried all these other therapies and would recommend them for help with hormonal problems.

- Acupuncture/acupressure
- Hands on healing
- EFT™
- Reflexology
- Aromatherapy
- Cranial sacral therapy

Chapter 10 :
THE EFFECT OF INFLAMMATION ON OBESITY AND ILL HEALTH

Inflammation is now being recognised as one of the main causes of ageing and obesity. Dr Nicholas Perricone, Dr Al Sears and Dr Joe Mercola, amongst others, have compiled masses of research on the subject. The conclusion is that inflammation is one of the major causes of ill health, ageing and obesity at the moment.

Their research shows that inflammation is one of the single greatest causes of aging and age-related diseases such as heart disease, diabetes, Alzheimer's disease, arthritis, certain forms of cancer, the loss of muscle mass and wrinkled, sagging skin – sounds awful doesn't it? It also shows that it is among one of the main causes of weight gain and obesity.

Inflammation is a very complicated subject and like the chapter on fats, I have to admit that I have rewritten this section about four times to get the right balance between the technical information and the key information that you need to know to reverse your own inflammation. I have decided to keep the subject as simple as possible and have only concentrated on the weight loss aspect, rather than include all the side effects of inflammation. If you want to know more I would suggest that you read Dr Perricone's books which are listed in the Recommended Reading List at the back of the book. His advice on anti-ageing is spectacular!

What is inflammation?

What is inflammation, anyway? Most of us are familiar with inflammation and have had it at some time of our lives. The classic signs are pain, swelling, redness, and heat like you get with a bad sore throat. However, this is good as the inflammation is a sign that your body is fighting the infection.

Inflammation is part of the body's natural defense system against infection, irritation and toxins. A specific cascade of events occurs in which the body's white blood cells and specific chemicals (cytokines) mobilise to protect you from foreign invaders.

But when the immune system is disrupted, it becomes inflamed and this inflammation then goes through the body very quickly.

It is therefore a vicious circle - being overweight promotes inflammation and inflammation promotes obesity.

As far as the weight aspect is concerned, we can track the changes back to the 80s when we were advised to eat low fat and high carbohydrates. In addition, processed foods such as white bread, snacks and crisps, became very popular. Even on the most sensible diet sheets they recommend cereal for breakfast, a sandwich for lunch and pasta with a tomato sauce for dinner – no protein in sight. You will discover in this book how important protein and fats are to losing and maintaining your weight and how wheat can cause weight gain and inflammation.

In simple terms, inflammation may be caused by:
- Eating a pro-inflammatory diet (i.e., high glycaemic carbohydrates)
- Environmental stressors
- Weakened immune system
- Excess exposure to ultraviolet light
- Hormonal changes
- Stress
- Alcohol

Diseases or illnesses caused by inflammation
- Arthritis
- Rheumatoid arthritis
- Cancer
- Obesity
- High blood pressure
- Heart attacks and strokes

Weight gain can be a side effect of eating pro-inflammatory foods
Our food selections are critical when it comes to causing and controlling inflammation. Foods that are pro-inflammatory, such as all forms of sugar and processed foods cause a highly destructive pro-inflammatory

response in our bodies. If we choose sugary or starchy foods, we trigger this pro-inflammatory release of sugar into our bloodstream, which causes our body to store fat rather than burn it for energy.

This causes acceleration of the ageing process of all organ systems in our body, including the skin, causing an increased risk of degenerative disease and inflexible, wrinkled, sagging skin and obesity. In addition, by eating that sugar, the resulting insulin response triggers our appetite, causing us to crave more and more of these types of carbohydrates, resulting in a vicious cycle of overeating.

After indulging in the wrong types of carbohydrates, in a matter of hours your 'feel-good' brain chemical, serotonin, will drop dramatically. These pro-inflammatory sugary, starchy foods will not only cause weight gain, wrinkles and fatigue—they will put you in a bad mood! - **and if you are suffering from PMS you can be assured that these foods will magnify all of the symptoms one hundredfold**.

Fortunately we can control inflammation in our bodies. It starts with the very foods we eat. All we have to do is avoid foods that provoke a 'glycaemic' response in the body, i.e. cause a rapid rise in blood sugar.

Avoid pro-inflammatory foods
Stay away from pro-inflammatory foods, which accelerate the ageing process. A simple rule of thumb is to consider the following - if it contains flour, and/or sugar or other sweetener, it will be pro-inflammatory. Sugary, starchy foods are poor choices and will not only pack on excess pounds but they will also make you look older than your years.

Bagels	Molasses
Baked goods	Muffins
Biscuits	Noodles
Breads, rolls	Pancakes
Cake	Pasta
Cereals (except old-fashioned oats)	Pastry
Chips/French fried	Peanut butter made with
Corn starch/cornflour	hydrogenated oils
Corn syrup	Pie
Crackers	Pitta bread
Croissants	Pizza
Doughnuts	Popcorn

Egg rolls	Potatoes
Fast food	Puddings
Fruit juice - eat the fruit instead	Rice
Flour	Shortening
Fried foods	Snack foods, including potato
Frozen yoghurt	crisps, pretzels, corn chips, rice
Granola	and corn cakes
Honey	Soda/fizzy drinks
Hot dogs	Tacos
Ice cream	Tortillas
Jams, jellies and preserves	Vegetable oils (other than olive
Margarine	or coconut)
	Waffles

The best foods to eat

Best protein choices (these are also rich in essential fatty acids, which help facilitate weight loss)	Wild Alaskan salmon, halibut, herring, trout, anchovies and sardines
Seafood choices	Shrimp, scallops, clams, mussels, crab, lobster, bass, cod and flounder
Best poultry choices	Skinless chicken breast and skinless turkey breast
Low fat varieties (if weight is a concern)	Plain yogurt, high essential fatty acid eggs, plain kefir, cottage cheese and tofu
Grains and legumes	Natural oats, lentils, chickpeas, dried beans, buckwheat and barley
Fruits and vegetables (The rainbow foods)	Apples, artichokes, asparagus, avocado, bamboo shoots, bell peppers (green and red), berries (blueberries, blackberries, strawberries, raspberries), bok choy, broccoli, Brussels sprouts,

	cabbage, cantaloupe melon, cauliflower, celery, cherries, chives, collards, courgettes, cucumbers, dark green leafy lettuces (baby greens), eggplant, endive, garlic, green beans, grapefruits (red and pink), honeydew melon, hot peppers, kale, leeks, lemons, mushrooms, onions, pears, pea pods, radishes, spring onions, Swiss chard, spinach, sprouts, summer squash, tomatoes, turnips, water chestnut and zucchini.
Nuts and seeds	Almonds, walnuts, hazelnuts, pecans, macadamia nuts, pumpkin seeds, sunflower seeds, sesame seeds and flaxseeds.
Herbs and spices	Cinnamon sticks, dill, marjoram, parsley, turmeric, ginger root, basil, oregano, thyme, lemon balm, mint, sage and rosemary.
Beverages	Green tea, water, Açaí (found in natural food stores), pomegranate juice (unsweetened).
Condiments	Extra-virgin olive oil (look for Italian or Spanish high quality), cayenne pepper, salsa.

To be healthy and maintain normal weight, we need all of the food groups - but not those that come from the laboratory. Our protein source needs to be pure, fresh (when possible) wild fish and other seafood, and free-range chicken and turkey that is hormone and antibiotic free. Our carbohydrates need to be fresh fruits and vegetables, preferably organic. And we need good fats, such as those found in salmon, sardines and other cold-water fish, extra virgin olive oil, nuts,

156

seeds, avocado, and acai berries (a Brazilian berry whose fatty-acid ratio resembles that of olive oil). These 'good' fats will help us absorb nutrients from our vegetables and fruits, keep our cells supple, our skin glowing and wrinkle-free, our brains sharp and our mood upbeat. We also need dietary fat to burn fat.

Dangers of inflammation

Cells respond to the way we treat them. If we keep them healthy and free of injury, if we give them the proper nourishment, they keep us alive and running at top form. If we don't, if we expose them to too much sun, to environmental toxins, to extended periods of stress, or to high-glycaemic sugars and starches, the cells will react by producing inflammatory chemicals as a deviation of the normal defence mechanism. And if we mistreat our cells in this way on a regular basis, we can end up with organ system failure and diseases like the ones listed, including metabolic syndrome, which can lead to diabetes and obesity.

This past decade has seen a complete turnaround in the way scientists regard white adipose tissue, better known as body fat. They no longer look upon it as an inert deposit of fat cells, stored as the result of overeating. They now realize that areas of fat storage are actually an active endocrine organ. Fat produces hormones, as do our pancreas, thyroid, parathyroid, adrenals, pineal, pituitary, and testes/ovaries, the organs that comprise the endocrine system.

I wish the doctors I had seen over the years thought this – all of them thought that if you were overweight you overate!

This is extremely important because the body fat itself controls how much body fat is going to be stored. It also affects our appetite, our energy expenditure, and our immune system. Body fat accomplishes this by secreting hormones known as adipokines. Adipokines are proteins that act as messengers throughout the body (more examples of the communications network). Like certain types of cytokines, those chemical messengers that have pro-inflammatory activity, adipokines can contribute to systemic, low-grade, chronic inflammation.

This becomes even more frightening when we begin to understand that the greater amount of fat we have stored, the greater its negative influence on the entire body, an extremely destructive, inflammatory influence.

Most overweight people, especially the obese, have chronic high levels of insulin that will begin to drop as soon as they start dieting. This is a two-edged sword, as low insulin levels decrease inflammation, which allows us to utilise body fat for energy. However, insulin is required to bring protein into the cells to maintain muscle mass. The overweight or obese person has cells that are insensitive to insulin due to their chronic high levels. That is, their body is so used to the overly high levels, it cannot recognise these new lower levels, thus it is unable to trigger the amino acid uptake needed to maintain muscle mass (insulin is needed to take up both sugar and amino acids into the muscle). This is why it is critical to take a powerful anti-inflammatory approach to dieting.

The effects of stress on inflammation
Stress is highly destructive - not just emotionally, but also physically. Unfortunately, in today's world, we all experience significant amounts of stress and it does not appear to be going away anytime soon.

Throughout this book, there is a detailed explanation of stress, cortisol and its effects. Cortisol is particularly damaging and causes inflammation.

Weight loss supplements that Dr Perricone recommends

These supplements not only help with inflammation but help raise the metabolism, aid fat burning and stops insulin spikes – in turn losing weight! These are available from Dr Perricone's website or from good health food shops. Full explanation will be found in the relevant chapters of this book.
- Caralluma fimbriata
- Chromate brand of chromium
- Maitake D-Fraction and SX Fraction Extract (a mushroom extract)
- Conjugated linoleic acid
- Carnitine and acetyl-L-Carnitine
- Alpha-lipoic acid Gamma linoleic acid
- L-glutamine powder
- High quality fish oil

Other supplement recommendations
- Gojii berry
- Acacia
- Turmeric

- Barley and Wheat grasses
- Astaxanthin – is a multifunctional antioxidant. This protects the cell membrane from free radicals
- I recommend Aloe Vera which is good for inflammation
- I recommend MSM which is good for joints (and makes your hair and nails grow)

Chapter 11:
YEAST OVERGROWTH AND CANDIDA

Do you have bloating, tiredness and crave sugar and carbohydrates? Added to that you can't lose your excess weight or you retain water? Then you could be suffering with yeast overgrowth of which candida is the most talked about form. This is almost at epidemic proportion, especially since we had been recommended to change our diet to more low fat high carbohydrates and less protein and most women have taken either antibiotics or the pill/HRT at some time of their lives.

Blaming everything on candida

When I first started investigating why I couldn't lose weight I went to a candida clinic. Their answer to every problem known to man was to do with yeast overgrowth and this is not correct. I am very wary of therapies that say they can 'cure' you, their therapy is better than anyone else's and that every disease from ME to thyroid to Parkinson's is caused by yeast overgrowth – because this is not true. It may be part of a problem but, as we know from my research, every problem has more than one cause and each cause has to be investigated separately.

When I starting testing myself, it turned out that I didn't have any yeast problem! This is why I specifically say in every chapter that you need to go to a therapist who has some form of testing or learn to test yourself. For example, my cravings were caused by hormones and imbalanced brain chemistry – not yeast problems. However, that is because I don't drink alcohol, don't eat sugar or carbohydrates and haven't taken antibiotics or the pill for years – so I wasn't a typical case.

However, when I swapped aspartame for sugar, I then developed a yeast problem in my bladder which proved very difficult to cure – especially as I wasn't keen to give up sugar in my tea as it was the only thing I had left that I really enjoyed. Because of the self-sabotage I couldn't take stevia or anything equivalent so I persisted with the sugar.

What is candida?
'Candida' is the popular term for an overgrowth of yeast - a condition known to medical doctors as 'intestinal candidiasis' when found in the

intestines or 'systemic candidiasis' when found elsewhere in the body. It was first diagnosed by American physicians in the 1970s.

Candida begins in the digestive system and little by little spreads to other parts of the body, normally via the blood stream. It is one of the main causes of thrush, so if you have recurrent thrush, yeast overgrowth is most probably the first place to start investigating why it reoccurs.

As I have said before, it is rife in the 21st century and is not recognised by the medial profession as a problem, especially not in the UK. Linked to the fact that it can show up as many different symptoms, it can be difficult to pinpoint and you may not be taken seriously by the medical profession but please do persevere.

What causes the overgrowth?
The damage to the intestinal wall allows toxins to enter the bloodstream. This condition called 'leaky gut syndrome' often leads to food allergies, foggy brain, migraines and depression. Symptoms in the intestines include diarrhoea or constipation, bloatedness, flatulence and itchy anus. Once through to the rest of the body, the candida can live anywhere there are mucous membranes - it particularly likes the vagina, lungs and the sinuses, providing food for bacteria and viruses. It has an ability to disrupt the endocrine system which can lead to weight gain or weight loss, PMS, menstrual irregularities, joint pains, asthma, hay fever, muscle fatigue and chronic tiredness. Testing usually reveals vitamin, mineral and enzyme deficiencies and low blood sugar. Thyroid tests often indicate that the thyroid is functioning normally, but body temperature is inexplicably low.

Some of the most obvious symptoms of candida overgrowth are thrush, cystitis and fungal infections of the nails or skin, such as athlete's foot. Local medication is not permanently successful. This list of symptoms is illustrative not exhaustive.

Many things cause the overgrowth of yeast but one of the main reasons is the increase in eating sugar and refined carbohydrates and the excess drinking of alcohol, especially wine – these are fatal combinations to get the yeast overgrowing.
- Use of antibiotics
- Alcohol, especially wine and beer with yeast
- The Pill and HRT
- Spermicidal creams and foams

- Steroids & other drugs
- Excessive carbohydrate and sugar intake
- Poor digestion
- Poor diet
- Dental mercury amalgam poisoning
- Chemical poisoning in the home or office
- Stress (usually as a contributory factor)
- Chlorine poisoning from tap water.
- Eating Foods to which you are allergic, such as yeast or gluten

Who gets candida?
Although men and children do suffer from candida, it is more of a woman's problem. Women seem to be more pre-disposed to this problem plus, of course, the oestrogen factor makes it worse and the female has one of the mucus membranes that the yeast love, the vagina, and that becomes thrush.

The candida diet
Recognise this diet? It is one recommended by some diet gurus as low fat and healthy but will promote yeast overgrowth, especially if you drink fizzy drinks and add a couple of pieces of fruit to the daily allowance:
  ✓ Cereal or toast for breakfast
  ✓ Sandwich for lunch
  ✓ Pasta with a tomato sauce for dinner

Can you see how this on a daily basis would lead to yeast overgrowth? Even if the bread is whole grain, there is far too much carbohydrate here and not enough protein. Added to this would be the sugar normally consumed during the day.
Symptoms of candida

The symptoms of yeast overgrowth are a bit like those of an under active thyroid – there are too many to mention! Listed below are the main ones but there is plenty of research on the internet which list all the symptoms that relate to yeast overgrowth.
- Absolute craving for food, especially sugar and carbohydrates. Sometimes the craving is so bad that it seems like there is somebody inside you doing the craving – well, there is! The yeast is doing the craving for the sugar and bread because it wants feeding.

- Irritability & mood swings
- Hormonal problems and PMS
- Bloating and wind
- Slow digestion and constipation
- Allergies, especially to bread and sugar, which makes the whole cycle worse
- Weight gain and oedema
- Immune system problems
- Aching joints and muscles
- Absolute tiredness and lethargy
- Foggy brain
- Thrush and cystitis
- Fungal infections of nails and skin
- Lose of libido
- Low thyroid or low adrenal function – in my opinion it is this that would cause candida not the other way around. If yeast overgrowth did manifest as low thyroid/low adrenal function it would be very mild

There is a mass of other symptoms as well and yeast overgrowth is thought to play a big part in ME and other immune system problems.

What to do to get rid of candida
The diet for yeast overgrowth has to be very strict at the beginning and I would suggest that you follow it to the letter for about six weeks and then review the situation – believe me the results will outweigh the pain of the diet!

- Cut out all fruits – I re-emphasis that the five a day should be mainly made up of vegetables and not fruit
- Cut out starchy vegetables, such as potatoes and parsnips
- Cut out all grains and that includes all bread – even the good-for-me-bread
- Cut out all other starches, such as pasta
- Cut out alcohol immediately and try to find an alternative to beer and wine in the future (beer and wine are full of yeast)
- Cut out mushrooms
- Cut out any food stuffs to which you may have an intolerance
- Cut out any food stuff that ferments in your digestive tract, like anything pickled

- Cut out all fizzy drinks
- Cut out all sugar and chocolate
- Cut out all artificial sweeteners – these should be replaced with Stevia
- Cut down your dairy consumption

After six weeks, start to introduce a piece of fruit a day and see if you get any cravings. If you do, withdraw all fruit for another few weeks and try again. It will be a trial and error situation and only you can determine which foods you will be able to end up eating. Please remember that alcohol is one of the worst things for you.

What food should you eat

- Lots of vegetables and salads (excluding starchy vegetables)
- Good quality protein – go for organic so you are not ingesting hormones or antibiotics from your meat or fish.
- Probiotic yoghurt which will help with the bacteria
- Add some nuts and seeds for vitamins and minerals
- Drink purified water

Alternative therapies

Colonic irrigation:
This is recommended but I am not sure about it! I used to have it and it made no difference whatsoever.

Reflexology:
This can stimulate the immune system.

EFT™
This technique is excellent for all sorts of reasons:
- You can relieve any symptoms especially for itching immediately
- You can start to reprogramme the body to stop the overgrowth of yeast
- You can explore the emotional aspects of candida. For example, if you get recurrent thrush you may have a problem with sex.

What herbs and nutrients can I take?

- Grapefruit seed extract – this has anti-bacterial, anti-viral and anti-fungal properties
- Garlic inhibits microbes, including yeasts and parasites
- Oregano oil is an excellent anti-fungi, yeast and parasite fighter
- Ginger promotes growth of good bacteria and inhibits bad bacteria
- Coconut oil/milk is brilliant as an anti-fungal
- Pau d'arco herb contains three anti-yeast compounds
- Acidophilus Bifidus – the good bacteria or any other probiotic is essential to get the balance of bacteria right
- Black walnut essence, which is also excellent for parasites and a metabolism booster
- Aloe vera juice will help the good bacteria settle in!
- Slippery elm which is excellent for digestive problems
- N-acetyl cysteine which boosts your body's production of the amino acid glutathione and has powerful healing effects.
- Zinc – this is very important for fighting candida
- Make sure you are having all your vitamins and minerals, especially Vitamin A, C & E
- B vitamins, especially Biotin

What homeopathy is available?

As you know I really love homeopathic remedies so dowse this list and see if any are suitable for you:

- Sulphur, which is good for digestive problems
- Sepia, which is excellent for yeast infection
- Natrum salicylicum, which is good for digestion
- Petroleum, which is good for mucus membrane and itching
- 6, 12 or 20c homeopathic potency of Candida albicans

New thinking and new research thinks that candida may be an endocrine disorder.

What is the APICH syndrome?

Autoimmune Polyendocrinopathy Immune-dysregulation Candidiasis Hypersensitivity syndrome – blimey what a mouthful! This syndrome was identified in the USA in the 1980s as an endocrine disorder afflicting all really difficult-to-treat candida patients and as discussed above it is far more prevalent in females. So it may be a good idea to dowse this name and see if you have it.

How do our hormones affect thrush?

Let's look at how our hormones affect thrush. The endocrine system governs the acid-alkaline balance in the vagina. Normally it is kept slightly acidic, but if the endocrine system decides to raise the pH level (making it alkaline), the vaginal wall becomes less hospitable to the bacteria that live there. They die, and the vacated space is filled by an organism that likes an alkaline environment i.e. thrush. This is why to get rid of thrush permanently, you need to return the vagina to its natural acidic state. Go gently - drastic treatment will certainly banish the thrush but a sudden vacuum will be quickly filled by an opportunistic strain of bacteria that will bring as many problems as the thrush. You also need to discover why your endocrine system is altering the acid-alkaline balance (e.g. are you taking HRT or other corticosteroids?) and let the body get back to the balance that it wants to maintain for your good health.

Other endocrine examples

When reading the above research I wonder if the endocrine system is responsible for a lot more cases of candida than we think. It is a well-known fact that candida may cause low thyroid and adrenal function but I feel it is also the other way around – a low thyroid and adrenal function cause candida and then it is nearly impossible to get rid of it. You also have the other organs of the endocrine system such as the pituitary, the pineal and hypothalamus, all of which have functions that affect hormones and the balance of the body.

When you are doing your diagnosis and self-testing using either dowsing or muscle testing, I would suggest that this is one of the questions that you ask: "Is my endocrine system causing my candida?"

More information

New information about candida is coming out all the time so why don't you do some more research on the internet?

Section 4

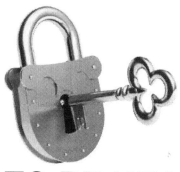

HOW TO BE HEALTHY
FOR LIFE

Chapter 12:
YOU ARE NOT ON A DIET, YOU ARE ON A HEALTHY EATING PLAN FOR LIFE

There are many, many diets on the market and they all offer amazing results. Impressive scientific reasons are given as to why this diet is better than another and this makes it very difficult to choose one. When you speak to most people who have tried unsuccessfully to lose or keep the weight off, they have tried all of the diets at one time or other. Also, the minute you consider a diet, the only thing that is on your mind is food, food, food and if you can't eat a particular food you become obsessed with it and then end up eating as much of it as you can!

I discuss in this book all the reasons why people can't lose weight or maintain their weight loss but eating is still a major part of this and of being healthy. It has been proven that diets don't work and when people have lost weight and then go back to their old eating habits they put the weight back on and in most cases more. Whatever you decide to do, it now has to be for life and you need to adjust whatever plan you chose to suit your needs and your life style. This doesn't mean that you can never again have a piece of cake, it just means that you have to allow for it in your daily calories or cut down the next day. You must work out what are going to be your coping strategies for handling special dinners, birthdays and holidays as this is for life. You need to investigate how you can make your diet interesting at all times because boredom is one of the reasons that people go off the rails. Do you add herbs and spices? Do you use EFT^{tm} to change your beliefs about food so that you eat more vegetables and fruit? Do you need to buy some new cook books? If you do much sure they are not the chefs cookbooks because they will add weight to you so please stay clear! Use your intuition, ask your guides and angels and imagine how interesting your food will be every day!

Most people miss the point of dieting which is also to cut down on portion size and to shrink your stomach to expect less food. I have heard of people eating as much as they can on their diet, for example a whole chicken on the Atkins or a Slimming World Red Day or 11 bananas a day on the banana diet. This is not educating your system to eat less, lose more weight or to start to enjoy the healthier things in life. It is just overloading your digestive system and making you want to eat more.

Both Al Sears and Joe Mercola, my favourite US doctors, both recommend cutting down on portion size and calories as this has been shown to prolong life and cause you less inflammatory degenerative problems.

People are said to be waiting for a pill so they can eat what they like. But then they may be slim on the outside but they will still have fat on the inside, around their vital organs, and this will shorten their life expectancy. Everybody needs to start eating things that are good for them.

In my opinion, the calorie charts of 2,000 calories for a women and 2,500 calories for a man were set before we had central heating and cars and when we were much more active than we are now. I think we all eat too much and generally need to cut down and use smaller plates and smaller portions. This is also because we were brought up to eat everything on our plate; otherwise we would get into trouble! In the UK they are revising the number of calories a day required and the amount is, I believe, going to be much lower.

According to the medical profession, you have to save 3,500 calories to lose one pound and therefore you would have to eat an extra 3,500 calories to put on a 1lb. Anybody who has struggled with their weight knows that this is absolutely ridiculous. You can put on 3lb at one meal – and you certainly haven't eaten 10,500 calories. This may work with somebody who has an excellent metabolism and a certain body type but it certainly doesn't work for most people I know, especially me! You need to find your own calorie loss formula and a good way of doing that is to keep a food diary and when you are introducing different food back into your life you can monitor whether it adds weight or not.

Healthy eating, not yo-yo dieting

The emphasis should be on being healthy. I do feel that the scale charts used by doctors for height/weight ratio are totally out of date. When I was a small size 12, according to the scale it showed that I was obese which was absolutely ridiculous! It doesn't matter what you weigh but it matters how you feel and how healthy you are. Eating healthily might mean that you don't lose all the weight you think you ought to lose, you may be a size bigger than you thought but as long as you are fit and healthy – that is the important thing. We need to change our perception from 'thin is beautiful' to 'healthy is beautiful'. Whoever said that this thin look was attractive anyway? This also means that you are not continually beating yourself up for not losing the weight or worse, feeling a failure because you have gained some weight. If you do not eat healthily then you are setting yourself up with problems in the future. This could be weak bones or muscles, diabetes, arthritis or some other degenerative disease, heart problems and, of course, a constant battle with your weight.

Yo-yo dieting is one of the worse things that you can do and that's normally what happens when you try and reach a target like I did. If you don't achieve the target, for whatever reason, you go off the rails and put weight on, beat yourself up and then start the process again, which is normally harder this time to achieve. The whole cycle is perpetuating! But if you are a healthy weight and maintain that weight then that is fine.

I could have cheerfully throttled Wallis Simpson for saying that you can never be too rich or too thin – she set everybody up with unrealistic expectations and eating disorders to boot. I am not sure about the rich bit though!

As you are eating for life you need to be able to add certain foods that you really like into your diet – perhaps a piece of chocolate or a glass of wine – you can't deprive yourself for life – that is when eating plans totally break down. But you shouldn't be drinking every day or eating chocolate every day so perhaps have a day when you are allowed this and it is counted into your calories? You need to find what works for you. But if you are really serious about losing weight you need to ditch the alcohol as this makes you retain water, makes you hungry and upsets your blood sugar.

My diet experience

I have tried every diet on the market and even got thrown out of Weight Watchers and Slimming World for putting on weight. I have starved myself, eaten three meals a day, grazed or whatever the latest fad is. My husband lost three stone on the Atkins diet and I lost nothing. I have detoxed, done the Cambridge diet – in fact I have done every conceivable diet or eating plan under the sun and at most lost seven pounds.

The thing that really annoys me is that everybody has an opinion and has suddenly become an expert on dieting (as they eat chocolate and drink a glass of wine!). The number of people from whom I have had comments (especially those who should know better) is unbelievable, ranging from advising that I should eat breakfast, I should eat more and I should eat less.

When I was able to lose weight for a few years (as described in My Story), I devised a plan which wasn't healthy but it enabled me then to lose weight. I ate 500 calories on a weekday and slightly more at the weekend. To counteract the effect of the weekend (because whatever I ate then was stored as water in my body – sometimes by one small meal on a Saturday night I could put on 7lb) on a Monday and perhaps a Tuesday I would cut the calories lower and this meant that the excess water would not turn to fat. The main problem is that most people eat slightly more at the weekend, and unless you take immediate action, the excess water will become fat.

I became very clever at not eating - I would order a starter when I went out and eat only half. I would mess around with chopsticks to make it look as if I was eating and I was bulimic for about six months – but luckily that revolted me so the food I ate got less and less. I would go for days without food, go away for weekends and not eat a thing, and would never eat so much as yoghurt as I thought it was wasted calories.

Because of this restriction I still have problems today. I eat small portions and could drop a meal very easily. I can't drink and eat together, not even a juice as I find it is too rich. I like to eat early as I hate that full feeling, especially when I go to bed. I can't eat anything rich or fried as it makes me feel queasy and any alcohol immediately goes straight to my head. This, of course, makes me a very cheap date, as I don't eat much and don't drink!

Endocrine system problems

My experience has taught me that if you have an endocrine problem, especially with the thyroid, then diets don't work at all. Even Dr Atkins admits that. If you have dieted before you will find it gets harder every time as you deplete your amino acids, neurotransmitters, vitamins, minerals and fatty acids and your metabolism slows down.

That is why I never read slimming magazines any more as they consist of stories of people who eat 5,000 calories a day and then cut down to 1,200 a day and the weight drops off. Of course, if you eat that much and cut calorie intake down substantially your weight will reduce and this also perpetuates the theory that all people are overweight because they eat too much. Remember that thyroid problems are as common as one in four people and most go undetected. That's without all the other imbalances that can happen.

I have spent the last thirty years researching diets and eating plans and I give a brief explanation later in this chapter of the most popular ones that are followed around the world. As you know, I believe that everybody is an individual and one eating plan will not suit all. Also everyone should stop talking about diets and start talking about healthy eating plans for life. We need to change our perception about eating and using junk food as treats for our kids as this is sending out a totally wrong message.

When I work with a client, I will muscle test or dowse to ascertain the best eating plan for that client:
- How many calories are required per day
- Whether a particular type of plan will suit, or a purely individual plan
- How many meals a day should be eaten
- The breakdown of protein, fats and carbs that the meals should contain
- Size of meals
- The time of night that the latest meal should be eaten
- Whether the food is required to be raw, cooked or a mixture
- Any food intolerances the client has

I don't normally recommend particular eating plans but I do recommend the following and they normally form part of the eating plan that my clients follow.

The Hay Diet	The Hay diet is where protein is not mixed with carbohydrates. The principle is that all foods digest at different times so by not mixing these two, digestion is quicker and more thorough. If you do not eat potatoes with your meat, you halve the calories and that has to be good. Also this way of eating aids the body to be at its optimum pH balance.

	John Mills ate the Hay diet for fifty years, was a picture of health and lived to a ripe old age. One of my wonderful friends, Daphne, cured herself of arthritis completely within three months and had the energy of a forty year old when she was eighty.
Metabolic Typing	Metabolic Typing is recommended by Joe Mercola. It divides everybody into three groups. One group eats mainly protein, one group eats mainly carbs and one group eats a mixed diet of protein and carbs. I am a typical protein type but cut it totally out of my diet because I was brought up to believe that protein was fattening and the enemy. Once I started to eat small amounts of protein I felt so much better. I felt full, satisfied and the cravings disappeared. Remember this is not an excuse to eat large quantities of protein! You should eat three small amounts of protein a day not a whole chicken for dinner!
Eat right for your diet	This is similar to Metabolic Typing (although Joe Mercola would most probably kill me for saying this!) but works on different blood groups eating different types of food. • Blood group O is a protein type • Blood group B is a protein and beans type but should still avoid wheat • Blood group A is a vegetarian diet
pH balance diet:	I explain quite a bit about this in the chapter on 'Other reasons why you can't lose weight'. I feel that it is vital to good health to keep your body's pH level at a slightly alkaline level. You need to balance in your diet the acid foods (grains and proteins) with alkaline foods such as vegetables (another good reason for eating loads of vegetables). You will not

	lose weight if your body is acidic because the fat cannot come out of the cells and it is as simple as that. The other eating plans I have recommended are also concerned with pH balance which makes them individual but a good all-rounder as well.
Body type diet	In the chapter on 'Body Types' I talk at length about different body types and how they affect your weight. I would do an analysis of my client's body type and in recommending an eating plan, would include foods that were beneficial to their particular body type.
Low GI diet	You should aim to include more foods with a low glycemic index in your diet. Your body will digest these foods slowly leaving you feeling full for longer and allowing you to eat fewer calories without feeling hungry. Adding a low GI food to a meal will lower the glycemic index of the whole meal. Buy yourself a good book and ensure that as many as possible of your foods are low GI.
5:2	I think this is excellent for people who want to maintain their weight and haven't been on a diet for years. For two days you eat 500 calories of "good for you food" and then the other days you eat what you like They assume that people will then pick "good for you food" but in my experience that doesn't always happen! I know people with a gastric band that liquidize chocolate!! But it is a good, healthy eating plan

My other recommendations

- Don't eat just because it is a mealtime, eat only when you are hungry
- Use your intuition to see if you should eat 2, 3, 4 or 5 meals a day

- Eat very slowly and chew each mouthful
- Eat want you want otherwise you will feel deprived, just make sure it is within your allotted calories or cut down the next day
- Sit down to eat your meal on a proper plate with a knife and fork
- Stop eating before you are full
- Use a smaller plate/use a blue or purple plate as this is an appetite suppressant
- Join a slimming club if you need support
- Halve your normal evening meal
- Always leave some food on your plate
- Cut out all processed food, biscuits, crisps and anything with transfats in it
- Cut out juices and energy drinks – they are really bad for you. Did you know that a glass of orange juice could have 200 calories in it – eat the fruit instead!
- People say cut out low fat but I am not sure I agree with this – a skinny latte is better for you and you are not drinking it to keep you full!! I do recommend low fat mayo and salad cream as the full fat ones are soooooooooooo calorific
- Fruit should be eaten in between meals as fruit digests quicker than protein and this would interfere with digestion
- Eat some protein with each meal
- You need to take into account calories, whatever anybody else says, so reduce calories and fat
- Take a photograph of what you eat every day
- Get somebody to pay you to lose weight or do it for charity
- Make sure you surround yourself with slimmer people as we are now getting "fat blindness" as people think it is the norm
- Have all around the house pictures of how you look now and how you want to look
- Eat a different amount of calories every day
- Don't shop when you are hungry
- Clear up your cupboards of everything you will stuck into your mouth!
- Write menus for the week, plan your meals and shop accordingly
- Keep a food diary
- Don't drink large quantities of fruit juice and smoothies

- Drink ice cold water as it is supposed to raise your metabolic rate by 30% which means you will burn up more calories!
- Alcohol should be restricted as this will make you extremely acidic, it is high in calories and it may give you water retention
- Don't eat anything with artificial sweetener as that will make you hungry
- Don't eat the olive oil that everybody is recommended – it is 200 calories a tablespoonful. Take capsules instead or eat oil fish
- Eat the best you can afford – good quality protein and vegetables
- Plan when going out for a meal! You do not need 3 courses, bread rolls and butter at more than 5,000 calories a time!
- Eat before going to a party so you are not tempted by all the sausage rolls!
- Be aware of dairy products as they are very fattening – do you really have to put spread on your jacket spud or a piece of toast – especially if you are going to put something else on it?
- Love the food that you eat and really enjoy it!
- Cut down on microwave meals and takeaways or have a small kebab or a chicken tikka
- BE ORGANISED!!!
- If you can't do any of the above use EFT™ to change your views so you can!

I do have a funny story about using smaller plates. Somebody I knew has been to Weight Watchers for years and finds that being weighed every week helps her keep her weight down. Miss (as she calls the lady who runs the class) was talking about using smaller plates to cut down on food intake and how this would help weight loss. The next week, one lady told the class "I couldn't fit all my food onto my small plate so I used two small plates". Apparently she couldn't understand why the rest of the class fell about laughing! You can see where some people go wrong with their diets can't you?

Reducing calories

Scientific research is now showing that by reducing calories, people will live longer, have better muscle tone and be much healthier. By eating lots of vegetables and reducing grain intake you will automatically reduce calories but have a healthier diet because of the reduced insulin levels and nutrients coming from the vegetables.

Don't think that you have to eat 1500 calories a day or the equivalent – concentrate on reducing meal sizes and calories.

I am not convinced that reducing the calories automatically puts you in starvation mode as stated by many doctors. I am not sure that the metabolism is slowed down that much if you don't have an endocrine problem and all your vitamins, minerals, amino acids and neuro-transmitters are in top working order. If there is a starvation mode it is most probably connected to past lives.

If lowering the calories puts you in starvation mode, why do people with gastric bands lose weight? Why do celebrities lose weight? Why do anorexics lose weight? All these people restrict their calories dramatically but all of them have excellent weight loss results

Why you shouldn't snack

There is a fascinating book called *Fat Land* which shows how America became so overweight and this cites snacking as being one of the main problems. If you look at countries in the 3rd World where they don't snack on crisps, fizzy drinks and chocolate they don't have a weight problem. In France they didn't have a weight problem but now in some areas the children are snacking and are starting to become obese.

If you must snack make sure that it is a healthy snack. Once again it is our perception that a chocolate bar is nicer than an apple and we therefore need to change our perceptions. Be aware of so called 'healthy' bars – many of them are full of sugar and fat. Please remember that the 'slimming' field is a £multi-million industry and much of what is sold is termed as healthy when it is not.

Eating healthily

We need to educate ourselves and our children to eat healthily and not look at fast food as a 'treat'. I seem to remember J Lo saying she loved her body very much and so she didn't want to put cream cakes into it. This is such a better perspective and we can change our ideas using EFT™ and reprogramming the subconscious. We can stop the craving and the addictions to food, we can help heal the emotions that may cause cravings but this chapter is about eating well for the rest of your life.

- Stop eating crisps and other snacks
- Stop eating chocolate except a small amount of very dark chocolate
- Stop eating anything with trans-fats, ie biscuits and pastry,
- Stop eating anything with MSG, additives and food colourings
- Stop eating packaged meals
- Stop eating fried food
- Stop eating anything refined, like white bread and white rice
- Stop takeaways and junk food
- Stop cooking in a microwave which kills all the nutrients in the food
- Stop eating too many dairy products as they are highly calorific and can also cause mucus
- Stop drinking fizzy drinks, either diet or not, as both are as bad as each other but the sweetener makes them additionally bad
- Start eating vegetables and fruit (at least 5 portions a day – more vegetables than fruit)
- Start eating nuts and seeds (but watch the calories as they are high)
- Start eating good quality protein
- Start eating a small amount of whole grains
- Start eating sprouted vegetables
- Start steaming food to retain nutrients, rather than boiling
- Start drinking flat mineral water slowly throughout the day preferably not from a plastic bottle but in a glass bottle, or filtered tap water

Some people would think that 'healthy' food is boring. I watched a programme last night on Middle Eastern cooking and the food was so colourful, full of fresh goodness and looked very tasty. If you think that is boring you need to change your beliefs because what you are eating now is killing you.

Eating out

Why do people who eat sensibly go berserk when they go out for a meal or at Christmas? Why do people need to eat three courses? Where do they put it all? Alcohol consumption is increased as well. It astounds me every time I go out – how can people eat so much in one sitting and then virtually go to bed afterwards? Why are they eating their entire week's calorie allowance in one sitting?

If you do overeat you need to cut down immediately to stop the water becoming fat, otherwise you will pay heavily for that one meal, especially if you have a water retention problem (even PMS water retention).

But why overeat? Why can't you just have one course or two small ones? Why do you have to have a huge creamy pudding at the end? The strain you are putting on your liver and digestion is tremendous and you therefore normally end up feeling absolutely awful.

To maintain your weight and stay healthy you really have to crack this one and keep it under control – do you feel deprived if you don't eat everything on the table when you go out or at Christmas – if this is the case get tapping with EFT™ and reverse those thoughts. If not, tap and find out why you have to eat like this?

When I say that I have been out for a curry people always assume that I have eaten at least two courses with rice and naan bread, and make disapproving noises. When I go out for a curry I normally have a simple vegetable dish with no rice or bread. Fairly low in calories, tasty and nutritious – what more could you want? This also shows how judgmental people are.

Five portions of vegetables and fruit a day

The government guidelines are to eat as much as five portions of vegetables and fruit a day. You will notice that I put vegetables first as it is important to eat more vegetables than fruit.

Fruit is high in sugar and therefore is more calorific than vegetables and can raise your sugar level. Stay away from smoothies and fruit juices unless they are consumed in very small amounts. It is much better to eat the whole fruit and take in the fibre and the sugar is released slowly. When you drink a smoothie or a large glass of fruit juice you are literally putting a whole shot of neat sugar into your system very quickly. This can affect the teeth and can also raise your blood sugar level and I believe fruit juice is one of the contributory factors for Diabetes II becoming so common. Also the calories are pretty horrendous – eat the whole fruit instead as it is far better for you.

Eat multi coloured vegetables and fruits and vary them as much as possible. Try to use organic produce as much as you can although I know this can be difficult and a little more expensive. The way I love to use vegetables is in soup, good old bubble and squeak, roasted winter and summer vegetables and curries. This way I can use lots of different vegetables and mix them together. I have to confess that I am not keen on a plate of steamed vegetables, but make it into a curry or bubble and squeak – yum, yum! Find out what suits you and your palate. Adding spices or herbs increases variety and flavour without adding calories.

We are very lucky as we have a great variety of vegetables to choose from. One of the great innovations of recent times is all the different salad leaves. I now love to have a salad made up of spinach, watercress, rocket, herbs and other salad leaves.

This means that you have to be well organised and prepared which takes a little training (I am a Virgo so it comes naturally!) – if you have a problem with organization do EFT™ to identify why you have a problem and put it right.

Drinks

It is so important to sip flat mineral water during the day. Notice that I say sip. That is because if you gulp water down it will go directly to your bladder whereas if you sip it will go to your cells.

If you have a healthy system you will not require a large amount of water to keep you hydrated and I would suggest that you dowse to find out how much water you should drink a day. The general advice about drinking two litres a day is not right for everybody and this is why you should dowse to find out how much is right for you. However, as a person with a water retention problem I don't agree that you have to drink pints a day, supposedly to flush the water out. In my experience this water sinks to my calves, ankles and stomach making them swell even more and become rock hard which is rather worrying. It doesn't wash out the water retention as some people say but a reasonable amount (one large glass in the morning and afternoon) will keep your cells refreshed.

It is good to cut down on caffeine, so look for caffeine-free tea and coffee but still try to keep these to a minimum as both make your system acidic. Perhaps introduce some herbals teas (which you do get used to I promise you, as some of them seem rather strange to begin with!). I drink dandelion coffee which is absolutely delicious.

Fizzy drinks are an absolute no-no – even water. The non-diet ones are full of sugar and have a tremendous calorific content whereas the diet ones are full of sweeteners which are best avoided. They are also full of additives, colours, and caffeine. Did you know that fizzy drinks (especially those with sweeteners) make you hungry? It is because they raise your blood sugar level and your stomach is expecting something tasty to eat. They are now being linked to pancreatic cancer as well. They are really bad for you and your children and will make them hyperactive. We have all seen children on fizzy drinks become more and more hyperactive so it is vital that they are replaced in your children's diet with water, caffeine-free tea and juices (fresh not containing additives etc).

Stevia should be the only sweetener that is used. It is a South American herb which also regulates the blood sugar level, so you are sweetening your tea and stopping your cravings at the same time – sounds good to me! All white sugar (and preferably brown as well) should be cut from your diet and more importantly your children's diet. You can also use honey to sweeten your food with but only a small amount. Another sweetener to use which is safe is called Xylitol which is found in plants. The taste can vary dramatically between brands, so you may have to try several – I must confess to never finding one that I like and that is why I stick to Stevia.

The right type of fats

I cannot emphasize enough how important this is and I have a whole chapter on good and bad fats. But I still wanted to put the information in this section because it is so important. We all need these fats for functioning of the body and, in fact, without them you won't lose weight because they are part of the metabolic process. However, you do still need to look at the calorific content so if you are introducing a hand full of nuts or olive oil into your diet daily, you will have to make a calorific saving somewhere else. You cannot add a couple of hundred calories a day to your diet without consequence unless you have a good metabolism.

It is also vital that you put into your body the right kinds of fats, such as oily fish, advocados, nuts and the new oil that is being hailed as a cure-all which is coconut oil. You may think these are calorific but the benefits far out way the calories and you will find that you are not so constipated, your skin and hair will be much better and your joints won't creak!

Cutting out other oils is essential, especially when frying. You should only use palm, rapeseed and coconut oils for frying. When the other oils reach as certain temperature they become toxic (even olive oil) so not are you only adding a horrendous amount of calories to your body and you are filling it with toxic matter as well. It is the top chefs that have got everybody frying again and this really should be banned!!

A George Foreman grill is the best option for cooking meat and fish instead of frying and you get the lovely grill marks on the food as well.

If you have a problem with chips or other fried foods, use EFT™ to retrain your subconscious to cutting them out altogether – they are really a total waste of calories. Also you don't have to fry onions etc before adding them to soups and curries – I never do with mine and my cooking tastes delicious. If you need to have chips, there is a new machine which cooks them in very little fat, or cook your own in the oven with a spray of one calorie fat.

In Scotland they eat a lot of fried food, including deep fried Mars Bar (ugh!) and they have one of the highest rates of heart disease in the world, so this speaks volumes – doesn't it?

Cooking from scratch

Why do people always say it takes too long to cook from scratch? How long does it take to grill a piece of fish or boil broccoli?!! Have a day a week where you batch cook the food you love and then freeze it in single portions so you always have food. Always freeze what is left over to stop you eating it!!! Don't pick at food or snack – you have no idea how many calories you are consuming! Don't finish the kids food off – throw that away!!

People also say that they can't afford good food. If you cut out the crisps, biscuits and junk food you will have more money to spend on other food. This is also an excuse – I know that a lot of people who can't afford organic but go to one of the cheaper supermarkets now and buy their value range which is excellent.

Other eating plans that you could follow

Why don't you get your dowser out and work out which is the best one of these to follow for you? Why not take elements out of all the diets and combine them into your own eating plan? It is also a good idea to go to a club as this keeps you focused and weighed every week.

The Greek Doctor & Mediterranean Diet	This diet is based on Mediterranean eating which includes, fish, vegetables and olive oil. You will have to devise your own 'for life' plan.
Weightwatchers	World famous way of eating working on a points system so you don't have to count calories. Also has a plan for life which is healthy. Good because you have other people to spur you on and you now have apps on phones.
Jenny Craig	If you can't be bothered to cook try a diet that is already cooked for you and all you have to do is heat. This one seems to come out as best.
Slimming World	Again, a well thought out plan that is for life.
GI diet	Works on slow releasing food using the Glycemic Index. This is supposed to keep you full and not snacking. An excellent routine if you are a carbs or mixed person but not particularly good for a protein person.
South Beach diet	High protein and low carbohydrate. Good for weight loss and anti-inflammatory.
Zone diet	Specialises in managing insulin levels by balancing the basic food groups: 40%t carbs, 30% fat, 30% protein.
Cortisol diet	This is to balance the adrenals and stress.

Cambridge Diet/ Lighterlife	Low calorie shakes, bars and soups contain all the nutrients you require. A very low calorie diet.
The Rosendale Diet	Concentrates on the hormone Leptin which turns off your hunger switch.

My 'eating for life' tips

As I have been on a 'diet eating plan' for my entire life I want to share with you the tips and the routines that I have found work for me – try them and see if they work for you.

1. Be organised:

OK, I know I am a Virgo with control issues (shoes in colour order and spices in alphabetical order!) but organisation is the key. You must try not to be hungry as this is when things go pear-shaped.

I also have a saying – some things are worth getting fat over. Although this statement sounds horrendous as I don't want to be fat but I use it as a guide to what I eat. If I go to a buffet and nothing is worth getting fat over, I will have a little salad or soup – I don't eat for the sake of it or because it is there. If I go out for dinner and again there nothing I particularly want I will have a starter or soup as my main course and feel absolutely fine about it. This is how I operate most of the time and I don't feel deprived in any way shape or form. However, if there is something that I really want I eat it and thoroughly enjoy it.

- Cook larger portions and freeze
- Always ensure that you have snacks and fruit available
- Always make sure you have your five veg and fruit available
- Buy frozen veg (it is fresher than a lot of 'fresh' veg)
- Make your own bread so you know what is in it and freeze
- Never go shopping hungry
- Clear everything fattening out of your cupboards

2. It's the little things that count:

- Use a smaller plate and always leave something on it
- Chew slowly and taste every mouthful
- Stop before you are full because it takes a while for the full message to reach the brain
- Eat what you want on one day (if that works for you)

- Cut back before, during or after if you are going to have a splurge
- Don't eat by the clock
- Don't watch the television or read when you eat and don't eat on the run
- Order a starter as a main course
- Don't hit the bread basket in a restaurant
- Don't hit the jacket potatoes as by the time you have either added a filling or butter they become extremely calorific

3. Drinking:
- Cut down on fruit juice and smoothies – eat the fruit instead
- Limit alcohol to the bare minimum
- Drink water every day, preferably a glass before each meal
- Don't drink fizzy drinks under any circumstances and that includes fizzy water
- Try not to drink too much when you are eating as this dilutes the stomach acid required for digestion

4. Other help:
- Carry round small bottles of salad cream and balsamic vinegar so you don't have super calorific dressings with salads – I always take my extra light salad cream on holiday with me (and if I go somewhere like India I take mango chutney as well – much to everybody's amusement!)
- Don't tell people you are on a diet as I am sure some force you to eat!
- Don't eat late and don't eat carbs after 6pm
- Don't eat fruit with a meal but in between meals
- Buy scales that show you various values like fat content or weight water points
- Keep a journal and tot up your day's calories (even if it is rough it is better than leaving it to chance)
- Don't listen to other people's advice. Usually they don't know what they are talking about.

5. Treating yourself:
I know that all this can sound a bit daunting but you must have a plan for rewarding yourself:
- Plan a non-food treat every three or four days, such as a manicure or buying something you really like

- If you can't live without a particular food or you must drink wine, decide how you are going to fit it in, once a week or eat as much as you like on one day?
- If you do have something that is not healthy, don't beat yourself you – look at why you wanted it.

Remember, when you look at food ask if this worth putting on 7lb for?

Studies

For a television program in the UK they took two very healthy young girls and fed one seven bars of chocolate a day and one junk food. Within a week the girl who was fed chocolate had put 7" on her waist. She had come out in spots, felt ill and, although she was a swimming champion, was finding it very difficult to swim at all. The girl on the junk food diet could barely get out of bed and felt so ill that she had to come off it in a week.

Somebody I used to work with drank an incredible amount of wine (she was always complaining of liver and kidney pain which would have worried me witless). When she decided to stop drinking and lose some weight she lost 5" from her midriff and 10lbs in one week – this shows how alcohol is stored around the middle and also adds to the water retention.

I really don't think that people realize just what damage junk food and alcohol is doing to them.

Conclusion

As this is going to be your eating plan for life you need to decide what you are going to do and how you are going to do it and stick to your plan. Of course, there will be times when you eat more but then you will have a plan of action to compensate, either by saving up your calories (this doesn't work for me) or cutting back immediately afterwards (this is the one that worked for me).

You need to be well organized and prepared – you will need to prepare snacks and lunches to take to work and to always make sure you have your five vegetables and fruit every day, with some good quality protein. There are no excuses for not being organised!

You owe it to yourself, your body and your children to take care of yourself, so start now and this will be the first day of the rest of your life! If we don't do something soon there will be whole generations that die early – and you don't want to be one of them.

I hear all the time that I don't have time for losing weight, cooking, exercising and anything else that is needed for weight loss. THIS IS JUST AN EXCUSE AND A DELAYING TACTIC – use EFT^tm to heal the need to procrastinate!

Chapter 13:
EXERCISE FOR LIFE

Everybody has to get moving more – that includes adults, children and pets! This is an exercise plan for LIFE so it must fit in with your lifestyle and above all it must be fun otherwise you are not going to do it. I hate gyms with a passion and find them very boring. I only like swimming in a hot country where I fall into a pool or the sea to cool off. So there is no point in me going to the gym or swimming for my exercise because I won't do it. Therefore I need to find something that excites me and that I want to do – and believe me there are plenty of different options.

When I had my beauty salon with toning tables (which were, by the way, a very good way to exercise but went out of fashion), I discovered that people have a funny attitude to exercising. Some people thought that they just needed one course and that would last them for the rest of their lives. Some people gave up for two months over Christmas and three months over the summer, so this undoes all the good they have done the rest of the year. All sorts of excuses were given as to why clients didn't keep their appointments. People are very fickle and would then go off and try something else or stop exercising at all.

I don't necessarily believe that you have to exercise to lose weight – when I was exercising for three hours a day it made no difference at all. I also have friends who can lose weight without exercising just by following a plan or cutting calories. I also am not really keen on boot camps – I feel that doing six hours of exercise a day is more likely to cause injury and you need time for your muscles to relax and heal.

But exercise makes you feel better, tones your muscles, helps your heart and your well being so you need to fit some exercise into every day.

What if you don't want to exercise?

We have mentioned changing your perception from negative to positive numerous times throughout this book by using EFT™. So if you don't want to exercise you need to find out why and use EFT™ until all those objections have been flattened. You then use the same techniques to reprogramme your subconscious to love exercise and want to include your exercise schedule in your daily routine, as effortlessly as cleaning your teeth. If you feel your motivation wane, get tapping again. Remember this is for life, not just a quick tone up.

Dowsing and muscle testing

You must be on the move and it has got to be fun and something you want to do. There is a lot of different information and most of it conflicts. Some say you should exercise every day, some say you should leave a day in between for the muscles to recover. The new information says you can exercise for nine minutes a week. Who do you believe and what is right for you that you are going to do it for the rest of your life?

This is where dowsing and muscle testing come in handy to ascertain what are the best exercise routines for you, how often and for how long should you do each one or. From this you can devise your own plan and you need to mark it in your diary a month in advance to ensure that you keep to your schedule. As shopping needs planning in order make sure you have the correct food in at the right time, so exercise time needs planning - mark the time out in your diary now otherwise it will get full up with other things. This is another clever self-sabotage mechanism!

Body Shapes

In Chapter 5 I talk about body shapes and how different shapes require different diets and different exercise routines. It is a good idea to check which body type you are and which exercise routines would suit you best and give the greatest benefits. Don't let this stop you doing what you want to do, just include in your week what is good for your body shape.

Other exercising

Please don't forgot that walking, house work, gardening, running upstairs, cycling and playing with the kids is all good exercise. Dancing round the living room is also wonderful exercise and great fun – and you cannot be stressed whilst you are dancing to Madonna letting yourself go. I love it (although the dogs find it rather strange!).

Start to build in other routines into your day. When you are waiting for the kettle to boil or in a queue, clench and release your bottom muscles

(I know you may get some funny looks but after you have been dowsing in a supermarket nothing fazes you!). When you sit at your desk make sure that you devise an exercise routine that you can do twice a day which relaxes the shoulders, ensures your posture is good and tightens the tummy and bottom muscles.

Use every opportunity you can and you will find that these routines become automatic. Look at a cat and a dog – when they get up they stretch every muscle. This is so good for you, too, so watch what they do and copy them. Animals have so much to teach us.

Why must you exercise? You need to exercise regularly for the following reasons:

- Burns calories
- Tones muscles
- Builds stamina
- Makes you feel better by releasing the feel good hormone
- Releases stress
- Releases anger
- Releases excess water
- Gives you a sense of achievement
- Gives you loads of energy
- Good for the heart and the circulation
- Good for water retention
- Good for bone density
- Good for burning fat
- Good for weight loss
- Good for cellulite

Exercise need not be expensive and most can be done in your own home. You don't have to join expensive gyms or have a personal trainer as you already have the equipment you need. Notice when you take the car on a short trip when you could walk, take the lift when you could use the stairs, take a walk at lunchtimes instead of sitting at your desk and just generally get moving. In the UK they recommend 10,000 steps a day which is quite a lot but to check out what you are doing buy a pedometer and see what else you need to do to reach the 10,000 steps.

People say they haven't got time to exercise but everybody watches the television and this is a good time to do your exercises. I have a supply of various devices bought very cheaply that I use whilst watching the television such as weights, a wheel for the tummy, a waist twister that you stand on, a tummy crunch machine, a device for putting in between your knees to tighten your inner thighs and doing all this normally lasts for one episode of Coronation Street!

You could get up fifteen minutes earlier in the morning to do some exercises but don't exercise last thing at night because this could keep you awake. So please, no more excuses! If you find exercising a bore then you need to change your attitude towards it so that you look at the positives that it gives you. For example several of my friends hate Sunday night because they have to go to work on Monday morning. I love Sunday nights because it is my pamper night when I have a face pack, manicure and pedicure and I really enjoy it. Can you see that I have changed my attitude to positive rather than negative? If you do this you will love exercise, not make any excuse not to do it!

Endocrine problems and exercise

As we have talked about many times in this book if you have a problem with your endocrine system, especially your thyroid, you will not burn as many calories or have as good muscle tone as people who have endocrine systems that work perfectly. So don't be disappointed or down hearted if you put in a lot of effort and don't see much result.

At one stage of my life I was exercising for nearly three hours per day. I was doing an hour on the toning tables, an hour walk with my beloved Jack Russell, Oliver, and either an hour's aerobic exercise class or a stepping class. On top of that I was doing yoga, callanetics and weights. You would have thought that I would have had a stream-lined body and lost weight but I didn't. I didn't increase my stamina either and every class was as hard as the last one. I did say to somebody once "why can't I lose weight with this exercise" to be told that if I did stepping four times a week the weight would drop off. Another bit of advice from somebody who didn't know what they were talking about!

So don't get disheartened because it is important for your heart, your bones and your circulation and once your thyroid is sorted out you will begin to see other benefits as well.

Cardiovascular exercise

This gets your heart going and should make you sweat. You should aim to do something like this three times a week for at least 20 minutes – this will obviously be adjusted for your body type and what the results are of your muscle testing.

- Walking
- Jogging
- Rowing
- Tennis
- Squash
- Badminton
- Dancing
- Housework
- Gardening
- Running up and down stairs
- Stepping
- Swimming
- Aerobic classes
- Trampolining
- Boxing
- Martial arts
- Cycling

Walking I have dogs and I love walking so this easily fits in with my lifestyle and it is also good for my dogs. If you haven't got a dog borrow somebody else's as it makes it more fun with a purpose. Walk in a beauty spot and not along the road side if you can which is far more pleasurable and you can convene with nature at the same time. There is a charity called the Cinnamon Trust where you walk dogs that belong to the elderly or people that have gone into hospital, so you could really feel as if you were making a difference as well as doing your exercise.

To turn walking into a full exercise, make sure you move your arms as well. Swing them as you walk and from time to time, if you can, lift them above your head and circle them.

Dancing Another of exercise I love is dancing so either take up a class or push back your furniture, put on your favourite record and dance to your heart's content and see how much better you feel. There are various dance classes around including salsa, ballet, ballroom, pole dancing but my favourite is belly dancing. Unfortunately belly dancing classes are difficult to find these days which is a shame because, not only is it good fun (in fact, it's absolutely hysterical when you first start) but also because the area that you are working on improves your sex life no end!

Gym

If you like going to the gym make the most of their equipment like running and rowing machines and steppers. I believe they also have new cycling classes called Spinning which involves using a bike (sounds like hard work to me!). Get a specialised plan for what you want to achieve and make sure that you make it as fun as possible and that it includes weight training suitable for your age and fitness. Take advantage of any of their classes and swimming pool which makes the gym membership better value and will encourage you to go more often. Go with a friend and make it a social occasion as having an exercise buddy keeps you going back for more.

Al Sears' PACE programme

Al Sears, who has been a hero of mine for many years, recommends his exercise plan called PACE into which he has put years of research. PACE stands for "progressively accelerating cardiopulmonary exertion" and it gradually challenges your heart, lungs, and blood vessels to build their strength. It involves doing short bursts of exercise with a resting phase between each burst. I have bought his book and I have to say that it has increased my stamina and muscle tone. He believes that short bursts with a resting time do far more good than an exercise such as jogging.

Other people are beginning to recognise that these short bursts are really helping with toning, weight loss and health and I now use this programme all the time. It is now being called HIT which stands for 'high intensity training' (how original!). Since starting this book, this form of exercise has become the favourite and has proven results – so this is one I would highly recommend.

A recent BBC program showed that after a month of three minutes a week exercise the doctor who was the guinea pig had less fat in his blood, better management of insulin and various other benefits. This one is definitely worth a try.

Vibrating Plate

As I am writing this the vibrating plate is the latest new toy which has been recently used by Madonna before her world-wide tour. What is it? It is a device that you stand or sit on to do your usual exercises and it vibrates. The plate works by giving the body muscles a high speed workout, as the vibrations make them contract and relax up to fifty times a second. Therefore you can give the body an hour's work out in fifteen minutes which sounds good to me.

I have just purchased a home use vibrating plate from ebay for a very reasonable price of £199, whereas the types for commercial use are anywhere between £2,000 and £6,000. Although mine isn't as powerful or as big as the commercial ones, it suits my needs (and my available space) perfectly. If you want to buy one, look around for the best deal before you do. You can place it in front of the television if you want to encourage yourself to use it.

I find it excellent and always use it whilst watching the television. However, if I were to buy one in the future, I would not buy one with a centre pole as when you want to lie on the plate, the centre pole gets in the way.

Jogging

I have always hated jogging and the excuse I use is that I have tiny feet for my height so I fall over a lot– believe it or not I really do, so jogging is not the best exercise for me. However, if it suits you it is a good all round exercise and a good calorie burner but make sure that you carry water, that you have the correct shoes on and that you jog somewhere beautiful – not by the road where you are breathing in all the exhaust fume. A jogging buddy or a jogging club is another tip to keep you on the straight and narrow.

If you feel silly jogging (like me!) start off by going round your garden and remember the Boy Scouts' method of jogging – jog for 20 paces and walk for 20 paces alternately.

Housework and gardening

Make your housework and gardening part of your exercise plan as anyone will tell you what hard work this is! Also running up and downstairs is wonderful exercise so every day, apart from normal activity, make a point of running up and downstairs twenty times a day in one go and feel your heart pounding. I have a three storey house and running up and down stairs with the ironing to the airing cupboard is great.

Stepping and aerobics classes

When I had my beauty salon my customers deserted the toning tables for stepping and in the middle 90s this was the most popular exercise going – although it could be a bit dangerous. Routines on the step box got so complicated that you spent more time concentrating on the routine and that's when injuries were caused by people falling off. However, I still think it is an excellent form of exercise so I purchased a step from ebay at a small cost. I had forgotten how great it was to do and it is another form of exercise that you can do at home in front of the television. I don't do complicate routines but I concentrate on pure stepping.

Swimming & aqua aerobics

If swimming is your thing then that's great. Swimming is a good form of exercise and if it is in a lovely pool it makes all the difference. For extra fun, join an aqua aerobics class. They make exercising slightly easier as the water takes the weight.

Remember to vary your strokes because solely using breast stroke can put pressure on your back and neck, (especially if you hold your neck out of the water like a turkey – this is what I do and end up with a stiff neck).

Trampolining According to Gillian Mckeith who wrote *You are what you eat*, jumping up and down on a small trampoline is the best aerobic exercise you can get. Apparently Gillian keeps a small one in a cupboard in her office that she gets out and uses in between clients. I have bought a small one which I use outside and she is definitely right – although it took me a little while to get used to using it.

Weight bearing exercise for healthy bones Weight-bearing exercise such as walking, running, tennis, weight training and aerobics are the best forms of exercise to help reduce bone loss associated with ageing. It is good to work with weights.

During these activities you are supporting your weight and so strengthening the bones. They then react to the forces exerted on them by becoming stronger.

These types of activities actually stimulate the osteoblasts, the cells which produce new bone tissue. For example, for the spine, an aerobic exercise class two or three times a week appears to improve bone density by 2-5%.

Remember you don't have to go to a gym but you can buy weights for home use. Repetition is the key, so if using weights aim to do three sets of eight to twelve repetitions but remember to build it up slowly.

Toning and stretching exercise

I have to say this is my favourite type of exercise without a doubt. I particularly love yoga and although Pilates can get quite advanced, I use a simple version to improve my core strength and keep my pelvis in line.

You can either go to a class for these particular toning and stretching exercises or you can buy a DVD and do them at home – personally I love throwing myself around the living room floor!

I enjoy the following exercise methods and do a combination of all of them as I think variety is good for keeping you keen and interested and you work on different muscles. You can do these routines every day and it helps with relaxation as well.

Types of toning and stretching exercises that I recommend highly:

Callanetics   About fifteen years ago I used to love callanetics and really felt the benefits of toning areas that I had never been able to tone before! Then, like toning tables, callanetics seemed to go out of fashion. Well I want to resurrect callanetics and feel that it is a very important part of weight loss and exercise which is aimed at reshaping the body – and it really does work. I do my callanetics watching the television, on holiday and in hotel rooms – it is totally portable and I love it!

Yoga   Yoga has been practiced for many thousands of years and has brought millions of people major benefits. To begin with it is better to go to a yoga class so you can understand the philosophy, the breathing and the relaxation which go together hand in hand.

Yoga is about stretching and strength whilst breathing properly. You do see some funny positions but don't be put off by that as you only need do what you are able to do - with an added bonus of a fifteen minute relaxation at the end of the session!

I do yoga every day and once again it is portable and suitable for holidays and hotel rooms. I have even been to places where they did sessions every day as part of the holiday.

My husband and I were once in an elephant retreat in northern Goa and the proprietor announced that we were all getting up the next day at 6am to do yoga before we went back to our hotel. Everybody started coming up with excuses but he was very insistent and even sent round his staff to wake us all up. He had a wonderful, simple routine that everybody did for about forty five minutes. The comments at the end – my asthma is better, I can breathe more easily, I can move my neck and loads more besides. Even my husband enjoyed it and felt better. All these people became converts; they were more relaxed and stress levels plummeted (although you are not stressed in Goa – one of my favourite places in the world!)

Pilates

Pilates is another wonderful form of exercise which bases its routines around your middle so it protects your back and tones your muscles, especially your pelvic floor muscles. Pilates is also portable to holidays and hotel rooms. It can be used in conjunction with resistance bands and balls (which can be used for other exercises apart from Pilates)

Toning classes

There are lots of exercise classes and DVDs that have specific routines, such as tums and bums and tops of arms (or bingo wings as we would call them!) I would suggest that, whatever your weakness, you have a DVD that mirrors your problem and do it every day. If you find it difficult to motivate yourself at home the best thing is to join a class.

A lot of people with flat tummies do a hundred sit-ups a day, perhaps that is something you would consider doing. It's best to do it when you get up in the morning before you leave your bedroom (otherwise you might not do it and escape!)

Oxycise

Oxycise is a very powerful breathing system, combined with flexing and contracting all your major muscle groups - anyone can do it anywhere, so once again it is portable to your holiday or hotel room. The Oxycise routine lasts for fifteen minutes, using oxygen which is essential for burning fat and revving up the metabolism. The exercises are simple to do and anybody of any age so can it so it is excellent for more mature people or those with limited mobility.

Tai Chi and Qigong   As well as yoga, it would be beneficial to include one of these into your weekly schedule. They are great for balance and calming the mind.

Toning tables   If you can still find a set of toning tables and you are over 40 I would suggest that you use them. They are a fantastic way of supporting any problem areas like backs whilst toning your muscles with resistance so they are excellent for bone building as well. I would like to buy a toning table to use at home but unfortunately don't have the space at the moment but as soon as I do I will buy one.

Facial exercise   We exercise the rest of our bodies but we forget our facial and eye muscles. There are various DVDs and exercise routines that you can do every day and I would recommend you do this even if you are having treatment with a face lift machine as the extra facial exercises will support the treatment you are having.

Some use extra devices that you place in your mouth and I have tried these and they are very successful. Eva Frasier is well renowned for her facial routines although they can get a little complicated with gloves and Vaseline!

There are free facial exercises at www.ageless.co.za.

I have found some interesting exercise to do if you have Bell's palsy at www.bellspalsy.ws/exercise.htm as you don't always have enough strength in your face to do the other exercises.

I found a brilliant device on Ebay which is a little machine that you put under your chin and it has a spring and you push your chin up and down – it has made the world of difference to my jaw line.

Children

Your children need to get active from a very early age and they must be encouraged to keep active. Once this is ingrained in them it becomes part of their life. Get them to help with the housework and gardening – there is no reason why they can't! It is most probably more important than ever with children these days spending too much time indoors at sedentary hobbies. Encourage your children to follow your good example. Why not join activity clubs as a family? These are just a selection of the activities/clubs you and kids could become involved in:

- Rugby
- Tennis (or other racket games)
- Football
- Athletics
- Netball
- Hockey
- Gymnastics
- Family walks, with or without dogs!
- Martial arts like Judo (and this also teaches discipline)
- Trampolining (but remember to have a side cover on so nobody falls off!)
- Cycling
- Playing

Pace Yourself

Don't go too mad at the beginning and then burn yourself out. You have to build up your stamina, so start slowly and don't be too hard on yourself. Remember, this is for life so don't put yourself off when you have just started!

If your muscles ache be sure to look after them and don't over assert yourself. Make sure that you always warm up and cool down as you don't want any injuries.

Vitamins and minerals

Make sure that you have enough vitamins and minerals that are required specifically for bones and muscles:

- Calcium

- Coral Calcium
- Zinc
- Magnesium
- Fish Oils
- Glucosamine in various different forms

Music and other distractions

To make exercise more fun, listen to your most stimulating music or watch your favourite soaps. You will find that the time whizzes past, just as the ironing does when we adopt the same idea (who would want to iron without the television on?!)

Remember your holidays

Even though you work hard all year on your exercise routine, it is surprising how all this hard work goes to pot once you are on holiday or away for a weekend. Your muscle tone can be lost during that fortnight so it is essential that some of your exercise routine is transported on your holidays with you, that you allow time during your day for it. If you make it part of the holiday, you also make it more enjoyable.

That's why the toning exercises are so good as you can do them in your hotel room or on the beach. You can also incorporate walking, running, swimming and cycling to ring the changes.

Don't forget sex!

Don't forget that sex is one of the best exercise routines you can have and burns lots of calories, so get snogging!

And the latest thing

Can believe that I have just purchased a pair of flip-flops called 'FitFlops' that exercise the legs as you walk (yes, I know there is one born every minute and it is usually me!). There are also trainers that exercise your muscles as you walk. I have a pair but I have found a problem in so much as if you have an issue it accentuates it and makes it worse, ie they affected my crooked pelvis so I only wear them a couple of days a week.

Doing it for you

There are various exercise machines that stimulate the muscles to contract that do the exercise for you. I have a Slendertone that I use at home and if I were going on holiday I would most probably pop in to my local beauty salon to have a few sessions to give me a boost.

In an old television programme on vets, the vet told a client that her Pekinese dog needed to have a daily walk to lose weight. The client reported back that the dog was having a wonderful walk and the vet was so pleased that he popped by to see the walk in action. To his amazement the butler was walking the dog on a velvet cushion, no less! The client got a telling off and the Peke, much to her disgust, was walked round the grounds on a lead (still by the butler I might add!). The moral of this story is that you need to do the work for yourself and only rely on these machines for a bit of a boost. As my mother would have said, "No pain, no gain" so get dirty and sweaty and begin to enjoy it!

There is always something new!

Every time I research part of my book there is always a new type of exercise that is being heralded as the future and the best ever. You need to use your discernment to see what type of exercise is best for you – sometimes the old and trusted methods are the best.

You don't seem to be any better?

In a recent program on the BBC showing the benefits of HIT, they also showed evidence from DNA samples that exercise doesn't benefit everybody. They call these people 'A fitness non-responder' and this would explain how some people (like me) never seem to gain stamina or good muscle tone. But this is not an excuse for not exercising.

Chapter 14:
FATS THAT HEAL, FATS THAT KILL

Once again, this chapter has been re-written about four times in an attempt to position the information at the right level to make it interesting and informative without being too technical or boring and if you would like further information about the many aspects of fats in more detail, I would suggest you read the several books listed in the Recommended Reading appendix or look at the masses of information on the good old internet.

Good fat, bad fat

With all the conflicting information available, you may be confused by all the hype about what fats you should eat and which ones you shouldn't eat. In the 70s and 80s, a food pyramid was developed which recommended a low fat diet to prevent such conditions as obesity, high cholesterol, heart disease, diabetes, and stroke. People therefore cut most of the fat from their diet, unfortunately cutting out the good fat as well. Surprisingly enough, obesity levels have spiralled and heart attacks and strokes are on the increase as well – so perhaps cutting the good fat out of your diet is not the best option.

Despite common misconception, not all fats are bad. Good fat does not cause obesity; instead, it's the excessive consumption of refined carbohydrates, sugar and all the other food types we have talked about in this book – especially processed food with hidden, unhealthy fats.

'Good' fats are **crucial** for good health and you must start including them in your diet **now**. The human body cannot survive without fat, since many body processes rely on fat, especially the thyroid and the metabolism. Yes, it is true that there are some fats that are not good for you. Not surprising, these **bad fats**, also known as trans-fats, primarily exist in heavily processed foods and they also contain many empty calories that you don't know about.

Eating **good fats** will make you fuller quicker and that feeling lasts for a long time. They are also very good for your skin and will help to stop you burning in the sun. They will stimulate your brain and your metabolic processes which also help with the feeling of well-being.

Good fats
Saturated Fats:
Saturated fats come from animal meat, dairy products and tropical plants (such as virgin coconut oil). These fats have come in for massive criticism and have been blamed for the increase in cholesterol and obesity. This is not entirely true – some saturated fats are good for you – in fact coconut oil is being hailed as the latest 'super food' and can help boost the metabolism and is ideal for cooking.

You need saturated fats for:
- For calcium to be effectively absorbed, at least 50% of dietary fats should be saturated
- Protecting the liver from alcohol and other toxins
- Enhancing the immune system
- For the proper utilsation of essential fatty acids

Unfortunately, saturated fats and trans-fats tend to be lumped together into one category as bad for you. Margarine contains trans-fat and butter contains saturated fats so it is better for you to eat butter – but do watch the calories.

You should get your saturated fat from sources like eggs and lean meats – not sausages and bacon!

BUT REMEMBER, EVERYTHING IN MODERATION!

Unsaturated Fats:
Studies have shown that unsaturated fats help decrease inflammation, reduce heart disease and boost the metabolism and are crucial in weight loss. It is now recognised that unsaturated fats lower the bad cholesterol (LDL) and increases the good cholesterol (HDL). The two types of unsaturated fats are polyunsaturated and monounsaturated fats.

Polyunsaturated fats are liquid at room temperature and they include corn oil, fish oil, flaxseed oil, hemp oil, pumpkin seed oil, safflower oil, sesame oil, soybean oil and sunflower oil.

Polyunsaturated fats are divided into two types: omega-6 and omega-3 oils. In the past we have all consumed far too much omega-6 (by eating more refined omega-6 oils such as soy, corn, sunflower and safflower oils) and far too little omega-3 which is derived from mainly oily fish, fish oil supplements and nuts and seeds.

Monounsaturated fats are also liquid at room temperature. They include olive, peanut, avocado, and canola oils. Olive oil and virgin olive oil are now used in most households. In fact, instead of putting a low calorie dressing on a salad, people are now mixing their own salad dressings with virgin olive oil and balsamic vinegar. Some people are starting to cook with olive oil as well.

Bad fats
Trans-fats:
Trans-fatty acids are produced when vegetable oils are heated under pressure with hydrogen and a catalyst, in a process called hydrogenation. Therefore, these fats are often referred to as hydrogenated or partially hydrogenated oils – so please study your food labels carefully.

Food manufacturers have added trans-fats into processed foods to prolong their shelf life and to replace saturated fats (which had a bad press) to make their products seem to be healthier for you. There is now a multi-million pound industry based around trans-fats. Manufacturers are realising that they have to withdraw trans-fats from their products – but watch out for what they are being replaced with. Another reason to cook your own food from scratch!

Trans-fats are commonly found in processed foods including pre-prepared meals, margarine, crisps, biscuits and crackers, most snacks and fried foods.

Below is a list of the generally accepted reasons for not eating trans-fats and you can see why trans-fats are being blamed for obesity and heart problems:
- Trans-fats cause weight gain and affect the metabolism
- Trans-fats lower good cholesterol and raises bad cholesterol
- Trans-fats can increase blockages in arteries
- Trans-fats affect blood insulin, increasing the risk of diabetes, diabetes II and Syndrome X and also makes you hungry
- ~Trans-fats cause inflammation

What are essential fatty acids (EFAs)?

The word 'essential' is used because they are a substance our body cannot produce and we must get these essential fatty acids from outside (from food or supplements).

The essential fatty acids are two of the most important of all the essential elements, ranking right up there with protein, as protein and the EFAs work hand-in-hand with each other. EFAs are the building bricks of our health and of your metabolism.

There are two families of EFAs: Omega-3 and Omega-6. Omega-9 is not included in this because the body can manufacture a small amount on its own, provided essential EFAs are present. This sentence is very technical but very interesting: "The number following "Omega-" represents the position of the first double bond, counting from the terminal methyl group on the molecule. Omega-3 fatty acids are derived from Linoleic Acid, Omega-6 from Linoleic Acid and Omega-9 from Oleic Acid" – just in case you wanted to know!

What do EFAs accomplish in the body?
EFAs support most of the body's processes, especially the metabolism and a good working endocrine system and these we are particularly interested in. They are also needed for growth and development in children.

EFA deficiency and Omega 6/3 imbalance is linked with serious health conditions, such as heart attacks, cancer, insulin resistance, depression and obesity. All of these illnesses are now spiralling out of control, with the most worrying being depression in children, for which vast amounts of anti- depressants are being prescribed.

**IT IS ESSENTIAL THAT YOU GET
YOUR QUOTA OF EFAs DAILY**

How Omega-3s aid weight control

Omega-3 (Linoleic Acid)
Alpha linoleic Acid (ALA) is the principal Omega-3 fatty acid, which a healthy human will convert into eicosapentaenoic acid (EPA), and later into docosahexaenoic acid (DHA) – now stay awake and read the next bit! EPA and the GLA synthesized from linoleic (Omega-6) acid and are later converted into hormone-like compounds known as eicosanoids, which aid in many bodily functions including vital organ function and intracellular activity and:

- Reduce inflammation that promotes weight gain
- Enable burning of dietary fats by transporting fatty acids into the mitochondria of our cells for burning as fuel
- Increase the burning of body fat
- Turn off the enzyme that creates body fat
- Improve blood sugar control by sensitising our cells and enabling receptors to respond to even small amounts of insulin.
- Stimulate the secretion of leptin, a peptide hormone that is produced by fat cells. Leptin acts on the hypothalamus to suppress appetite and burn fat stored in adipose tissue (fat cells)
- Influence key anti-obesity genetic switches

Found in these foods:
Flaxseed oil (flaxseed oil has the highest linoleic content of any food), flaxseeds, flaxseed meal, hempseed oil, hempseeds, walnuts, pumpkin seeds, Brazil nuts, sesame seeds, avocados, some dark leafy green vegetables, canola oil (cold-pressed and unrefined), soybean oil, wheat germ oil, salmon, mackerel, sardines, anchovies, tuna, and others.

Omega-6 (Linoleic acid)
Linoleic Acid is the primary Omega-6 fatty acid. A healthy human with good nutrition will convert linoleic acid into gamma linoleic acid (GLA), which will later be synthesised, with EPA from the Omega-3 group, into eicosanoids. This greatly improves PMS and hormonal water retention, together with other diseases such as arthritis. It is also great for the skin and skin disorders like psoriasis and eczema.

Found in these foods:
Flaxseed oil, flaxseeds, flaxseed meal, hempseed oil, hempseeds, grape seed oil, pumpkin seeds, pine nuts, pistachio nuts, sunflower seeds, olive oil, olives, borage oil, evening primrose oil, black currant seed oil, chestnut oil, chicken, plus many others

Corn, safflower, sunflower, soybean and cottonseed oils are also sources of linoleic acid but are refined and may be nutrient-deficient

Omega-9 (Oleic acid)
Oleic acid is essential but technically not an EFA because the human body can manufacture a limited amount, provided essential EFAs are present.

Monounsaturated oleic acid lowers heart attack risk and arteriosclerosis, and aids in cancer prevention.

Found in these foods:
Olive oil (virgin or extra virgin), olives, avocados, almonds, peanuts, sesame oil, pecans, pistachio nuts, cashews, hazelnuts and macadamia nuts, etc.

Eicosanoids
When Omega-6 and omega-3 fatty acids are metabolised, they produce eicosanoids, which can have dramatically different effects on your body. The omega-6 fatty acids found in processed food and vegetable oil products produce 'bad' eicosanoids and the Omega-3 fatty acids found abundantly in cold water fish and fish oils produce 'good' eicosanoids, which control silent inflammation.

I have included eicosanoids in this chapter because you may feel that all eicosanoids are bad for you and they are not.

Supplements
Choose which of these oils to take every day:

Fish Oil   A fish oil supplement should be taken every day – this is normally in the form of Omega 3 as the majority of people have too much Omega 6. It's great to have oil in your diet but if you have a problem with your weight you cannot suddenly add 200-300 calories a day without making adjustments elsewhere, otherwise you will put on weight – not what we want!

In the UK, a group of twelve year old children were given fish oils every day. After two months their reading ability had gone up by two years – fish oils are now given out in some schools everyday as part of the school day and if I had children mine would definitely take fish oils.

Because of awful diets, mainly consisting of processed or junk food (especially in children) and the fact that suntan lotion is extensively used so we don't get exposed to enough sunlight, vitamin D levels are very low. This is another reason for taking fish oil (cod liver oil) as it will boost vitamin D levels as well as all the other benefits.

Also don't forget to eat oily fish at least twice a week and if possible eat free range/organic fish. Salmon, tuna and other oily fish are best but eat what fish you like as often as possible.

The omega-3 in fish is high in two fatty acids crucial to human health, DHA and EPA. These two fatty acids are pivotal in preventing heart disease, cancer, and many other diseases. The human brain is also highly dependent on DHA - low DHA levels have been linked to depression, schizophrenia, memory loss, and a higher risk of developing Alzheimer's - this makes sense as depression and other problems are rising dramatically and more and more children are being prescribed medication for attention disorders.

Flaxseed oil Some people prefer to take flaxseed oil instead of fish oils and obviously if you are a vegetarian this is the best way to take your daily oil supplement.

Flaxseed oil contains alpha-linoleic acid (ALA) which helps in the conversion of Omega-3 to DHA and EPA.

Most of the research available has been done with fish oil and not flaxseed so you will see the benefit of fish oils recorded, but not necessarily the benefits of flaxseed.

One advantage is that you don't get that awful 'fish belch' when you take flaxseed oil!

Sancha Oil Al Sears has just started selling a new wonder Omega-3 product called Sacha Inchi Oil which comes from South America

Sacha Inchi is the vegetable species with the highest concentration of Omega-3 on the planet; it has a high concentration of proteins, vitamins A & E, and essential amino acids.

Sacha Inchi Oil is taken orally (2 teaspoons a day) or can be consumed with salads. I always have a bottle handy but must confess to putting mine on salads rather than off a teaspoon!

Evening primrose oil (or equivalent) Evening primrose oil contains substantial amounts of Omega-6 which in turn gives you the EFAs that you need. In addition to Omega-6 fatty acids, evening primrose oil contains linoleic acid and gamma-linoleic acid (GLA). Both linoleic acid and GLA are believed to have very positive health and medicinal indications. Linoleic acid may affect how the body utilises insulin, maintains weight, and fights cancer and heart disease. GLA may help to inhibit the body's production of chemicals that cause inflammation. Consequently, evening primrose oil has been used in connection with inflammatory conditions, including both rheumatoid arthritis and asthma. Some studies have also suggested that evening primrose oil may be useful in treating chronic fatigue syndrome but more research is needed before evening primrose oil can be recommended for that condition.

Evening primrose oil may help to relieve pre-menstrual syndrome (PMS), symptoms of menopause and breast pain due to hormonal changes during menstruation - I can certainly vouch for that one!

Vitamin E oil Take good quality Vitamin E oil every day. This is a powerful antioxidant and is excellent for the skin. Break a capsule and rub into your skin!

CLA Conjugated Linoleic Acid (CLA) is becoming a weight loss superstar because of its effect to promote fat-burning and enhance lean muscle growth. It comes from meat and some other saturated fat sources, so has been eliminated from many diets. It has also been shown to be anti-carcinogenic and anti-inflammatory, whilst it improves blood lipid profiles. In studies, CLA has been shown to have a powerful effect on reducing body fat and increasing lean body mass. I take this too, as I don't have any saturated fat in my diet and I don't eat meat.

Oils to use everyday

Olive oil The Mediterranean diet has long been held up as one of the healthiest ways of eating in the world and this is mainly due to the olive oil that is used. Olive oil is good for you and should be used in salad dressings – virgin olive oil being the best. Remember to take the calories into account if you are adding olive oil to dressings. However, olive oil is slightly toxic if it is used for frying, so use an alternative.

Coconut oil Coconut oil has many health-giving properties, amongst which is its conversion by the body into the hormone pregnenolone. It has important immune-stimulating and antioxidant actions, while it stimulates metabolism and increases thermogenesis (fat-burning). Substitute coconut oil for butter or margarine in cooking as a better, tastier alternative to either of those harmful fats. Coconut oil is also perfect for applying to dry skin or adding to bathwater. Coconut oil will become a solid at room temperature or any temperature below 74 degrees. Unlike other cooking oils, coconut oil does not become rancid. Be assured that coconut oil is cold-processed, non- hydrogenated, it contains no trans-fatty acids and it will not cause a rise in cholesterol levels. It does contain some saturated fat but in a good way.

Fat burning (Thermogenesis)

We all want to raise our metabolism to a safe level to help us lose and maintain weight. In the body, heat creation comes from the conversion of food into energy and the heat given off as a by-product of energy metabolism. We all know people who can eat what they like and remain slim (damn them!) whilst the rest of us struggle. This is where good fats come in because they help with this process.

Chapter 15:
HOW DEEP BREATHING WILL HELP YOU LOSE WEIGHT

You will probably be thinking what a peculiar chapter to have because we all breathe. However, the problem is that we don't breathe properly – we breathe very shallowly and we are not getting enough oxygen into our cells. Also most metabolic processes need oxygen too, so they will not be performing as well as they could and the main process that is affected is the metabolism. Now you are becoming interested!

A friend of mine who used a therapy called Buteyko to help her breathing, lost 7lbs in one month and she certainly wasn't dieting as she didn't need to lose any weight. Proper breathing techniques will speed up your metabolism, cause you to lose weight and make you feel better at the same time, including masses of energy.

Don't forget that you have to persevere and add these breathing routines to your daily routine, which will include meditation, visualisation and affirmations (amongst others).

What else can correct breathing do?

- Curb your appetite
- Eliminates waste and toxins which are stored in fat cells
- Make you more alkaline
- Feed your cells
- Improve your skin, hair and nails
- Kick start the lymphatic and circulatory system
- Kick start the metabolism and help with weight loss
- Energise the heart
- Controls binge eating and cravings
- Help activate the brown fat to burn calories
- Calm you down
- Reduce stress and anxiety
- Release emotions
- Make exercise more powerful with better muscle tone

- Give you more energy and stamina
- Can help problems like asthma, panic attacks and anxiety

Nose or mouth?

The question is, do I breathe through my nose or my mouth? The answer is that it depends on the type of breathing routine you do but during the day it is best to breathe through your nose. Buteyko suggests that you loosely put some tape across your mouth (especially at night) to stop you breathing through your mouth and breathe only through your nose. This is quite hard at first and needs practice but it does get better eventually.

I find that if I am doing deep breathing to calm down or in meditation, I prefer to breathe in through my nose and out through my mouth. But this is really down to personal choice or the method that you are using.

What is deep belly or diaphragmatic breathing and how do you do it?

The explanation from Wikipedia is as follows:

Diaphragmatic breathing or deep breathing is the act of breathing deep into your lungs by flexing your diaphragm rather than breathing shallowly by flexing your rib cage. This deep breathing is marked by expansion of the stomach (abdomen) rather than the chest when breathing. It is generally considered a healthier and fuller way to ingest oxygen, and is often used as a therapy for hyperventilation and anxiety disorders.

Performing diaphragmatic breathing can be therapeutic, and with enough practice, can become your standard way of breathing.

To breathe diaphragmatically, or with the diaphragm, one must draw air into the lungs in a way which will expand the stomach and not the chest. It is best to perform these breaths as long, slow intakes of air, allowing the body to absorb all of the inhaled oxygen while simultaneously relaxing the breather. To do this comfortably, it is often best to loosen tight-fitting pants/belts/skirts as these can interfere with the body's ability to intake air.

While at first one may not feel comfortable not expanding the chest during breathing, diaphragmatic breathing actually fills up the majority of the lungs with oxygen, much more than chest-breathing or shallow breathing.

A common diaphragmatic breathing exercise is as follows:
1. Sit or lie comfortably, with loose garments
2. Put one hand on your chest and one on your stomach
3. Slowly inhale through your nose or through pursed lips (to slow down the intake of breath)
4. As you inhale, feel your stomach expand with your hand. If your chest expands, focus on breathing with your <u>diaphragm</u>
5. Slowly exhale through pursed lips to regulate the release of air
6. Rest and repeat.

This may seem uncomfortable at first so practice, practice and practice! This will eventually become second nature. I must confess when I first started that I found it very difficult to do. This type of breathing is used with various exercise routines such as Pilates, Callanetics, Yoga and Oxycise to increase their power and fat burning or relaxation capabilities. You will get it but it does take time.

Basic breathing techniques

Triangle breathing	This is a simple exercise that you can do anywhere:

1. Simply inhale through the nose for a count of four
2. Hold the air in your lungs for a count of four
3. Exhale through the nose for a count of four

Do this exercise for three to four minutes at one go and notice the difference to your wellbeing almost immediately. If you can imagine a triangle whilst completing this exercise it will help with your focus and to keep your rhythm.

Square breathing	This is the same exercise as above but hold for four counts after the exhalation and then pause between taking in the next breath.

Make sure that this is part of your daily routine

and if you feel yourself using short gasps, centre yourself and do one of the above breathing exercises until you become calm and relaxed – this is brilliant for stress.

Kung Fu

Do 10 quick Kung Fu breathes before each meal – this really gets your digestion going!

1. Stand up
2. As you inhale deeply through your nose, tilt the head back as if you were looking for dust on a chandelier
3. Pause for a millisecond before
4. Exhaling forcefully through your mouth. Make a loud definitely "ha" sound as you bring your head back to its normal position

Baywatch Bikini

Do three sets of ten Baywatch Bikini breaths to get your metabolism fired up broken up into sets of ten (if you have three meals a day you will be doing more than thirty). Start the day with a set of ten and do another set of ten after every meal.

1. Stand tall and say out loud "I am the greatest" – mean it and feel it
2. Take a long deep belly breathe, inhaling through your nose
3. Lock the breath in your body and hold it for four times as long as you inhaled. For example, if you inhaled for a count of four, hold it for a count of sixteen.
4. Now exhale through the mouth twice as long as you inhaled. Using the example above, if you inhaled for four you exhale for eight.

Alternate nostril breathing

Believe it or not we breathe through different nostrils at different times of the day and we find it easier to breathe through one nostril than the other.

The right nostril energizes the left side of the brain which controls logic and verbal activity. The left nostril energizes the right side of the brain which controls creative activity. So use the technique for coordinating the left/right brain function.

Use right thumb for closing right nostril, right ring finger for closing left nostril

1. Close left nostril, inhale right nostril (4 counts) pause (8 counts)
2. Close right nostril, exhale left nostril (8 counts) pause (8 counts)
3. Keep right nostril closed, inhale left nostril (4 counts) pause (8 counts)
4. Close left nostril, exhale right nostril (8 counts) pause (8 counts)

Repeat steps 1-4

Breath of Fire

This breath cleanses the body and strengthens the lungs. As it creates heat it is good for anger and other similar emotions and eliminating thoughts.
1. Inhale
2. Using diaphragm, force air in and out in rapid repetitions with emphasis on the out breath
3. Inhale deeply
4. Exhale rapidly with force, pull diaphragm up and toward back
5. Pause
6. Take a few recovery breaths (normal breathing) before starting another round.

Repeat steps 1-6

Buteyko

A friend of mine who had asthma discovered the therapy called Buteyko which she used very successfully to control any attacks and she no longer needed her medication. She also lost about 7lbs with no change to her diet (which she could have done without as she wasn't dieting – typical isn't it?).

Buteyko works on the carbon dioxide mix in the body and advocates breathing through the nose as opposed to the mouth. For more information on this contact a Buteyko therapist or read *The Carbon Dioxide Syndrome,* which is fascinating.

However, I went to a talk about Buteyko and was told that it 'cured' weight problems – remember that not one single therapy can cure anything! Also, if I were honest, she talked 'at' me the whole time she was talking about weight (and eating) which rather put me off, especially as she was very slim but then proceeded to have an enormous lunch with alcohol and said she was off to eat and drink her way around France. You can see why she didn't impress me, can't you?

Section 5

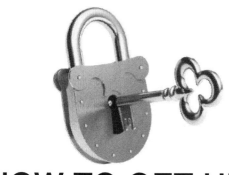

HOW TO GET HELP NATURALLY

Chapter 16:
HOW TO SUPRESS YOUR APPETITE

Introduction

If all your hormones, vitamins, minerals, amino acids and brain chemistry are balanced then you shouldn't need any appetite suppressants or other slimming pills as you should find that cravings are virtually non-existent and your metabolism should be functioning correctly. However there are times when you may need a little help (PMS, after a holiday or similar) so I have investigated what is available to you, both prescribed and alternative.

From my research and what is written in the papers, many people seem to have an enormous appetite and have trouble controlling what they eat. Appetite suppressants and techniques can certainly help in these cases.

There are masses of options available on the market and from my research I have picked ones of which I have had experience, friends have experienced or which have had good reported results. I had to cut this section down otherwise it would be confusing and over one hundred pages long! Some of these recommendations will also help to reduce fat but I have decided to put them in this section as they are also an appetite suppressant.

I also include other techniques that have been talked about in this book to reinforce how they can be used for appetite suppression and raising the metabolism. Remember that before you take any supplements you should get it checked with a practitioner who uses dowsing and/or muscle testing as a diagnostic tool. If in any doubt contact your doctor, as herbal remedies can affect prescribed medication.

I have listed homeopathy and herbs for weight loss as different chapters as they support specific organ functions rather than appetite.

A note on what can make you hungry, so don't do it!

If you do any of the following you will become hungry for various reasons:

- Chew gum (some people say this takes the appetite away but I find it increases it)
- Drink large quantities of fruit juice or smoothies
- Use sweeteners
- Eat sweets, including mints
- Drink fizzy drinks
- Drink alcohol in quantity – one glass is ok
- Smoke (smoking raises the metabolism by about 200 calories a day but this does eventually even itself out so don't use it as an excuse for not giving up!)

These either activate the saliva or raise the blood sugar level so that the stomach thinks it is going to receive food – which of course it isn't.

Explanation of herbs and homeopathy used

In the relevant chapters there is a full explanation of all the herbs and homeopathy that are contained in the prepared medication listed in this section, plus many more herbs and homeopathic remedies that are used in controlling weight, excess water and supporting the liver and any other organs.

Information changes so quickly

I was in our local health food store the other day asking for acai berries and the supervisor asked what they were. I replied that they were the 'latest thing' and would cure everything, including weight and would stop me aging! The poor lady replied "Blimey, last week it was goji berries – it is so difficult to keep up". I have to agree with her 100%. One week it is pomegranates that are good for you and the next it is mangosteen. It is all very confusing and this is where your diagnostic tools come in very handy because you can cut through all the marketing bumph and pick out what is especially right for you. I have included acai and goji berries in this section because I do believe that they have a large part to play in weight loss.

I have now drawn a line under any new products as I have to take a stand somewhere, although somebody is bound to point out that I have missed one! The supplements are listed in alphabetical order and not in order of importance. The ones I heavily recommend are marked with an '*'.

Prescribed appetite suppressants, such as Phentermine

I have taken these myself for several years and they were the only way I could lose weight at that time and they were teamed up with diuretics for maximum effect.

Therefore I couldn't possibly criticise anybody else for taking them as they do boost the metabolism slightly for the time that you take them. However, they come with lots of side effects, including addiction and, most importantly, they are not fixing the problem of why your metabolism may be so slow. These are really not the answer.

At the time of writing, there is a new wonder drug is called Acomplia, which claims to drop your body weight by 10%. Sounds fantastic doesn't it but it does it by reducing appetite so it is no different to any of the others. If you can't lose weight by dieting (ie you have cut your calorie intake down) how are these going to help in the long term? If you need something, please use a herbal alternative.

Herbal Alternatives:

Acai Berries***	These berries are supposed to speed up weight loss; zap wrinkles and boost energy levels. Dr Perricone (US skin guru) has dubbed the berries the 'No 1 anti-ageing food' so they are in my cupboard as well.
Adios	Adios speeds up the body's metabolism and works on burning fat. Adios contains butternut, dandelion root, boldo and focus. This is widely used in the UK with good results.
Caralluma fimbriata******	This is a herb from Bali that not only is an appetite suppressant but will help fill you up and lose weight. This is in Al Sear's Bali Slim and I use it and highly recommend it.
Elixir.com appetite	Elixir.com uses a mixture of homeopathic remedies which when combined make an

suppressants*	ideal and efficient appetite suppressant. It includes support for the thyroid and the metabolism as well.
Green Coffee	This is one of the latest appetite and weight loss products to hit the shelves. Helps curb the appetite and maximize weight loss.
Herbal Phentermine (as opposed to the prescribed Phentermine)	Herbal-Phentermine works to increase your metabolism, suppress your appetite, burn calories and increase energy.. It doesn't have Ephedra, Ma Huang, and Ephedrine which have been identified as causing problems with certain people. I haven't tried it myself but it has good reports and results.
HGC Injections/ Homeopathy ******	Over 50 years ago, a British endocrinologist Dr. Albert T. Simeons discovered the potential benefits of HCG injections while studying pregnant females in India. The popularity of HCG grew when noted author Kevin Trudeau began promoting the injections as a weight loss solution in his work *The Weight Loss Cure 'They' Don't Want You to Know About.*
	HCG stands for human choriogonadotropin and is a hormone produced by pregnant women. HCG has a wonderful effect on the human body in that, in small doses, it suppresses hunger and activates adipose fat tissues. A very low calorie diet is followed (mainly fish and vegetables) which actives the hypothalamus and this kicks in the body's ability to use its stored fat, especially around the middle. So the face still looks healthy and the person looks well and this

is maintained after the treatment is finished.

You can have either daily injections or take the homeopathy remedy. I, of course, prefer the homeopathy version and have taken this myself with excellent results.

I got mine from www.doeshcgwork.com/homeopathic - and yes, it does work.

Himalayan Goji Berries and Juice**

This juice has almost every vitamin and amino acid that is required for weight loss and because of this it reduces appetite, increases metabolism and encourages fat burning.
They have been nicknamed 'the cellulite assassin' by a top US dermatologist, which can't be bad. I am hooked on these berries but you only need to take 10g a day and no more, so don't eat the whole packet at once!

Honey, garlic and vinegar capsules***

HGV as it is called is now being hailed as one of the new weight loss miracles. It eliminates natural cravings for high fat foods and is supposed to double weight loss as part of a calorie controlled diet, as well as lowering your cholesterol and blood pressure.

Hoodia*****

This seems to be by far the most important and effective appetite suppressant around and is widely sold in various guises. I have tried it myself with amazing effects so I would highly recommend it if you need to suppress your appetite at any time.

The Hoodia Gordonii plant is an herb, which grows naturally in the harsh desert conditions of the Kalahari Desert of Southern Africa. For many generations the nomadic SAN tribe's people of the region have used the Hoodia Gordonii plant to suppress appetite and thirst during long hunting trips of several days duration

Although there are over 20 species in the Hoodia family only the Hoodia Gordonii plant contains a natural appetite suppressant.

A good product to have is the Hoodia Lollipops – I always have a couple in my handbag. Not only do they take away your appetite but they give you a tremendous boost of energy – which we all need!

Hydroxy Citric Acid***

Hydroxy citric acid is found in the rind of fruits specifically Garcinia cambogia, which is found across India to southeast Asia. HCA has now become extracted commercially and can be bought on its own and combined with other ingredients for a weight loss supplement. (Citrimax and Super Citrimax contain HCA).

HCA can inhibit the enzyme citrate lyase, which is needed for the conversion of carbohydrates into fat. Citrate lyase is only active when there is a high influx of carbohydrates in the diet, so inhibiting this enzyme will only be of benefit in achieving weight loss when consuming high carbohydrate content meals.
It may also suppress the appetite and increase your feeling of wellbeing – sounds like it would be worth a try.

Lipitrex

Lipitrex has other ingredients for slimming but the main ingredient for appetite control is called PinnoThin. PinnoThin is a natural ingredient, obtained from a special oriental pine tree nut, that can help stimulate the release of a hunger-suppressing hormone, so there's less chance you'll feel hungry. Recent research conducted on PinnoThin reveals that within thirty minutes of taking this supplement, people had less desire to eat and when they did eat, they ate significantly smaller portions. I haven't taken this myself but the reports and the results look good.

Metabolife Ultra

I have no experience of this but it seems to be very popular and have good results. The ingredients are quite simple, with various vitamins and minerals, especially chromium, which you already know is a good appetite suppressant. The other ingredients that are also used for appetite and slimming aids are Guarana and a patented Garcinia extract called Super Citrimax.

Pyruvate

Pyruvate is found naturally in the body and in foods such as cheese, red apples and red wine. It has been proved to speed up metabolism, is good for building muscle and is particularly good for burning fat. It is also thought to be an appetite suppressant.

Raspberry Keytone*****

This is the latest to help curb the appetite and lose weight and it has had very good reviews.

Slimthru

This is a new drink that is being marketed in the UK. It contains palm and oat oil which is supposed to keep you satisfied longer long. The idea is that these two oils stay for longer in your gut and that makes you less hungry.

Trimsecret

This 5-step plan has been formulated by Jan de Vries, the famous Dutch herbalist who now lives and works in Scotland (luckily for us because he is one of my heroes!). Trimsecrets are capsules that you take before each meal and contain vitamin C, citrus fruits powder, yerba mate, green tea extract, guarana, citrus aurantium powder, gum arabica and chromium polynicotinate.

Wheatgrass***

The juice of this plant is said to speed up tissue healing, cleanse the liver and helps stabilise blood sugar (which wards off sugar cravings). It has more appetite suppressing protein than chicken, eggs or fish and more iron than spinach. It is rich in a host of minerals and can be bought as a drink or in a capsule.

Other avenues to try

Minerals

In my opinion the best thing out for appetite suppression is the mineral chromium. You should take this every day and watch your appetite disappear!

Scent

Dr Alan Hirsch's idea for the SprinkleThin happened quite by chanced. He was treating patients with head trauma who had lost their senses of smell and taste and discovered that almost every single one of these patients gains between 10 and 20lbs. Could there be a connection? There was - and SprinkleThin was developed.

Why It Works
Even though SprinkleThin contains no fat, no

calories, no sugar and no stimulants, it seems to have a profound effect on the eating experience. Dr. Hirsch says: "I think that SprinkleThin works because it actually enhances the taste and smell of food as you eat. These 'tastant crystals' seem to affect the delicate chemosensory receptors in your nose and mouth. These receptors then signal the brain that you've eaten enough. Your brain starts shutting down your appetite and tells the body that it is satiated, or full." By eating less, your body is less likely to store excess calories as fat.

I can certainly recommend SprinkleThin, especially when you first start out and your stomach hasn't shrunk or your brain chemistry is not fully functioning. Also, please bear in mind that if you have an under active thyroid you will have very little sense of smell or taste.

I would certainly recommend SprinkleThin, certainly when you are cutting down in the beginning before your appetite and your stomach shrink!

Vanilla

I had a vanilla car air freshener and I was convinced that this affected my appetite as when I got to work I was never hungry. This was later confirmed in an article I read which said that vanilla was an excellent appetite suppressant when breathed in (as opposed to eaten). It's a good idea to burn vanilla candles (safely of course), use an aroma diffuser, have a vanilla air freshener in your office, home or car or have a room spray. This one is simple, cheap and really works! Make sure it is organic so that it you don't have an intolerance to it.

Patchouli essential oil

We always thought that the hippies were slim because of the drugs they took but in fact it could have been patchouli, which at that time was a popular essential oil! Patchouli has been proved to be a successful appetite suppressant.

Burn this as an essential oil or candle, or wear it as a perfume. You can also pop some in your bath. I can really confirm that it works.

Water

Remember, if you are hungry you may be hydrated, so always start by SIPPING a glass of water slowly. If you drink it too quickly it will just go straight through your system. It has to be water and not squash or a similar equivalent. Drink good quality water and preferably not out of a plastic bottle. Don't drink it too cold either, room temperature or warm is best. My grandmother had warm water to drink every morning when she got up and lived to be 90! The water should be still as fizzy water can cause weight gain and water retention.

Other techniques

EFT™

In the chapter on Emotional Freedom Technique (EFT™) we look at all the ways that this can help with losing and maintaining weight. It can also be adapted for cravings and appetite control very easily. All commands and instructions for EFT™ are listed in the chapter, so the following are just reminders of what you can do.

Affirmations for EFT™:
- Even though I am hungry, I deeply and utterly love and accept myself, I chose not to eat
- Even though I am craving crisps, I love and respect myself but I chose to go for a walk instead
- Even though I am stuffing my face because I am stuffing down my emotions, I love and accept myself but I choose to face my emotions and eat healthily

- Even though I am addicted to sweets because I have no sweetness in my life, I deeply love and accept myself but I chose to love myself and fill myself with that sweetness

Positive Affirmations
- I am full and nourished
- I am nourished physically, emotionally and spiritually
- My metabolism is burning up all my food and I am nourished

Self-hypnosis Self-hypnosis is a wonderful way of reprogramming your subconscious with new patterns and eliminating old patterns. There is a wealth of self-hypnosis CDs on the market. However, I highly recommend Paul Mckenna.

Subliminal PC software Subliminal messages are messages that are flashed frequently either onto a television or PC screen which help to install positive messages into your subconscious. I have some software installed at work which is flashing messages to me all the time. Do a search on the internet and buy yourself some weight loss subliminal software (or you may even get it free) – if you are going to sit in front of your television or computer you might as well make the most of it!

Remembering when you felt good about yourself This is a very simple and easy exercise to do and is excellent if you are feeling down or you are craving food. Sit quietly and remember a time when you felt really good and motivated. Let this experience wash over you and fill every cell of your body. Feel really good and smile to yourself and rub your finger and thumb together. This is anchoring this wonderful motivated feeling to this physical act. So when you are down, just about to grab food or need motivation, rub your finger and thumb together and remember that previous happy experience. Stop and really feel the motivation and how good it felt. By now you should be motivated not to eat.

Visualisation   You by now will have visualised the person you want to become or want to maintain. My person is a tall, slimish lady with long blonde curly hair and wears a red suit with high heels. This is how I looked when I felt my best. When I am down or my resolve is fading I think of my visualisation and keep it in my mind's eye, I imagine it and make it real and then I step into it. Draw a picture of how you want to be and put it on your fridge door, on your pc screen at work and in your manifest box or board. The good thing about visualisation is that it can be done anywhere and anytime.

Distraction   When a puppy is behaving inappropriately you are told to distract him by some method, perhaps by throwing a ball. You can try this method (not by throwing a ball though!) but thinking of something else, doing something else, walking into another room or something similar.

If you are hungry or craving food always wait ten minutes before you eat it and you normally find (unless it is PMS) that the craving or the feeling will disappear.

Good old fashioned willpower   People seem to have forgotten about all about this and it really does work. I gave up a forty a day smoking habit and only put on a 1lb. To me, to replace smoking with eating seemed a ridiculous thing to do so I organised myself to do something else with my hands – de-fluff my sweaters! It never occurred to me to start smoking again, having been through the pain of giving it up. So sometimes you just have to say NO! I AM NOT GOING TO EAT THAT and be strong willed. You will love yourself for it!

Other slimming aids

These pills don't necessarily fall into the appetite suppressant, herbs or homeopathy chapters. It also contains slimming products that use a combination of herbs and supplements. I especially like the ones that Al Sears sells.

Collatrim   Nature's Sunshine's team of research scientists has developed a new blend called Collatrim Plus. This liquid combination of nutritional and herbal ingredients supports weight loss and enhances the body's ability to burn fat
The ingredients are: Conjugated linoleic acid (CLA) may benefit weight loss due to its ability to increase metabolic rate and reduce fat storage. Collagen makes up one-third of mammal protein. Digestive juices and enzymes act on collagen, breaking it down into amino acids, which are then used to build lean muscle mass. L-carnitine boosts energy because it helps in the process of fat burning. Garcinia cambogia is good for weight loss and raising the metabolism.

Zotrim   Zotrim works by delaying the rate at which the stomach empties by an average of 20 minutes which makes you fuller for longer and therefore you eat less. It is also an appetite suppressant and works on raising the metabolism Contains Guarana, Yerbe Mate and Damiana.
The results that are logged on the internet look good, boosted by the fact that you are fuller for longer – which is always a good thing!

Al Sears   Bali Slim contains Caralluma Fimbriata which is the latest thing!! And it is called Bali Slim because it comes from Bali!
- Curcumin – an active component in the treasured spice turmeric, it's also *thermogenic*. It may help increase metabolic rate. Think of it like turning

233

up the heat in your cells – the temperature goes up and the fat is converted into energy. This may actually dissolve fat cells.

- Chromium – improves body composition by promoting balanced blood sugar levels, which may help control your appetite
- Caralluma fimbriata- its nickname is 'famine food'. Not only does it suppress your appetite – giving you the feeling of being satisfied and full – but it also increases endurance and quenches thirst. Instead of struggling to adhere to a strict diet, this cactus makes it easier for you to feel satisfied when you eat smaller meals

Primal Lean   This contains Irvingia Gabonensis which is thought to help leptin which helps you lose weight quickly and feel better.

- Chromium – improves body composition by promoting balanced blood sugar levels, which may help control your appetite
- Irvingia Gabonesis – an African herb which is called bush mango. This has been used for hundreds of years to fill the people who live in the bush up as they didn't know where their next meal is coming from
- Fucoxanthin – seaweed extract so helps with thyroid and metabolism
- Garcinia cambodgia – an Indian herb that helps with appetite and weight loss

Phenylethylamine   Phenylethylamine, also known as PEA, is both the name of a standalone product and an ingredient in many weight loss supplements. PEA is a stimulatory transmitter, which improves the mood of the user and increases alertness. It is derived from the amino acid phenylalanine. The supplement company, PrimaForce, markets Phenylethylamine as a dietary supplement that aids concentration and focus and enhances mood.

By stimulating the release of dopamine, PEA reduces appetite while improving mood.

Drawbacks and dangers:
Phenylethylamine's value as a weight loss supplement has not been substantiated by recorded studies. While the chemical occurs naturally in chocolate, it is also the brain altering ingredient in LSD and morphine. Excessive amounts of phenylethylamine could lead to psychoactive effects, such as hallucinations. In extreme cases, PEA can be lethal.

I haven't used this personally, but the results on the internet seem very good.

Fat blockers

These are supposed to take the fats straight out your system which means that the calories will be removed. However, this also takes the GOOD fat out of your body and as discussed in various chapters of this book, your body needs good fats. This process also removes a good deal of vitamins and minerals from your body as well. They also have various side effects like nausea and diarrhoea and can make you depressed.

I haven't personally taken a fat blocker but I have a couple of friends that have. I was told that it made them quite ill and not able to go very far from a toilet. They also said that they didn't lose any weight taking it so I'll let you make up your own mind on this. I wouldn't take it.

There is a natural fat blocker which is from a

cactus called opuntia ficus-indica and it reduces the quantity of fat that is absorbed. There are various companies that put this in capsule form.

Carb Blockers   It would be so much easier to limit your carbohydrate intake than use pills to block the carbohydrates you are eating. By now you should be eating healthily and your body needs the carbohydrates that you are eating to perform their functions, such as absorption of vitamins and minerals and as fibre.

Diuretics   Sometimes it is a good idea to take some form of diuretic to aid the loss of water, especially when you have PMS. There are a host of herbal remedies that you can buy over the counter which support the kidneys and the bladder, whereas prescribed diuretics don't. My favourite for getting rid of excess water is a homeopathic remedy called Apis Mel.

Keeping a check on your calories

Some people have no idea how much food they are eating, especially when they go out for a meal. Although calories are considered old hat now, I still find it helps to tot up the calories as it gives me a rule of thumb as to what I have had. The following suggestions help:

- Photograph your food - so that you see the plate as a whole – it may give you a surprise. Then put together all the photographs of the days food – believe me this curbs your appetite! Then put in on Facebook.
- Keep a food journal – this also gives you a clue as to times of day/month or other stresses that make you turn to food. This also curbs your appetite!
- Lay out all your day's food on one table, especially if you have lots of takeaways. I saw this done on a television programme and the result was shocking!

Other tips:
- Get paid to lose weight – this is an excellent way of motivating yourself – the old fashioned ways always work!

- Join a club of get together with friends or have an equivalent of an AA buddy who you can ring if you feel yourself falling back
- Don't tell people you are on a diet – you are not on a diet you are eating healthily for the rest of your live. Have plenty of excuses ready as to why you can't eat or drink certain things – it is so much easier if these replies are practiced. Don't let people bully you – I have been bullied for years for not drinking alcohol or eating puddings.
- Treat yourself every few days – buy something nice or have a massage. Start to give yourself 'non-food' treats.

New discoveries by the medical profession

All the time, the medical profession is developing solutions to the obesity problem by trying to curb appetites and for the body not to absorb so much fat.

I am may be cynical, but when you read the research it is normally based around lowering calories by lowering appetite or releasing the fat before it is absorbed. Work is now underway on devices that are put into the stomach, chewing gum and a vast array of other pills or potions that they hope will work. There is no doubt that there is a whole new multi- million pound industry at stake, as 'obesity' is the in thing and there is a shedload of money to be made from it – you only have to look at the diet foods available now and the new baby on the market 'smoothies'.

CRT - Device that fools the brain:
This is not really a therapy but a device to control hunger. British doctors are trialing the match stick sized device that is placed beneath the skin of the abdomen. This device is programmed by doctors to send signals activating the stomach's nerves which reduce the feeling of hunger.

As people don't always eat when they are hungry (three course meals, for example) this is not the answer. The answer is to change people's attitude to food.

Hormone Peptide Y:
Scientists at University College London and King's College London have been using brain scans and have identified the appetite regulating hormone peptide Y (PYY). It targets not only the primitive areas

controlling the basic hunger urges but also the pleasure and reward centres. PYY is released from the gut into the bloodstream after eating and signals to the brain that food has been eaten. A nasal spray containing the hormones is being trialed.

Chapter 17:
HOMEOPATHY FOR WEIGHT LOSS

What is homeopathy?

Homeopathy is a therapeutic system of medicine that is based on the principle of like-cures-like – which means that a substance that can cause certain symptoms in a healthy person can cure similar symptoms in an unhealthy person. Homeopathy aims to aid and stimulate the body's own defence and immune processes and is derived from a variety of plants, animal materials and minerals. They are prescribed to fit each individual's needs, are given in much smaller and less toxic doses than traditional medications, and are used for both prevention and treatment. Established two hundred years ago by German physician, Samuel Hahneman, homeopathy is now recognised by the World Health Organisation as the second largest therapeutic system in the world.

Homeopathy considers a patient's complaints in totality, viewing them as a whole - as an integrated entity - and not as a collection of body parts. So it treats the person or animal as a whole (called a 'constitutional' remedy). Homeopathic medicines are very effective in both acute (such as a cold) and chronic conditions (such as arthritis). Homeopathy treats health problems, personality and emotional issues at the same time, which is so important for the body to balance and heal itself.

Please remember that all medicine has contra-indications and may react with your prescribed medicine or with an existing condition that you may have. If in doubt, please check with your doctor or vet and then consult a qualified practitioner. If you don't wish to medicate your pet yourself, homeopathy for an animal can only be prescribed by a homeopathic vet, not by a homeopathic practitioner for humans.

What is a constitutional remedy?

A constitutional remedy is the remedy that homeopaths prescribe to eliminate all the problems that your 'type' may have in their lives, such as arthritis, cancer and other serious problems to which you may be prone. When you take this remedy you should find that it will automatically heal the areas of your body that are out of balance – these could be your thyroid, leptin and appetite problems or anything else related to weight/water gain such as a sluggish lymphatic system.

However, you could need additional remedies to sort out your appetite, get your kidneys going or boost your immune system.

I am going to compare two different remedies so you can see how homeopathy begins to work and how different these people are:

Calc Carb
Calc carb is made of oyster shells and is a remedy that is used in weight loss as well as other things.

This is a profile of these people (I am one of these):

Personality	Quiet, cautious and very sensitive. They can be anxious and worried and hate cruelty of any kind.
Likes	Sweet foods especially biscuits, sour foods, starchy foods, cold drinks and ice cream, eggs and oysters.
Dislikes	Milk and coffee.
Other features	May crave odd things like chalk and soil.
Fears	Fear of darkness and ghosts, incurable illness and cancer, death, enclosed spaces, thunderstorms, poverty and mice.
Physical appearance	Can have a healthy appetite which can lead to weight gain but are also slow and sluggish. Slow metabolism and water retention. Can be clumsy.
Weak areas	Weight gain, glands, throat, ears, nose, bowels and bones.

Phosphorus
This is a remedy that is used for anxieties and fears that can cause insomnia and exhaustions. Also used for digestive complaints, respiratory problems, bones and teeth. These people dislike being alone and like sympathy!

This is a profile of these people:

Personality They need lots of stimulation to give their imaginative natures a boost so they don't become irritable. They love to be the centre of attention.

Likes Salty food, spicy food, fizzy drinks, sweet food, cheese, ice cream, wine.

Dislikes Fresh fruit, tomatoes.

Other features They are upset by hot foods and drinks, and milk.

Fears Darkness and ghosts, burglars and being alone, thunderstorms and water, failure in business, illness, cancer and death.

Physical appearance They are usually tall, slim and well proportioned. Their skin is fine and pale and blushes and flushes easily. They have either fair or dark hair with a coppery twinge. They dress with flair and flamboyance.

Weak areas Bones, teeth, lungs, left side of the body, nervous system, circulatory system.

Where to buy the remedies

Homeopathy can be bought from Boots or Holland & Barratt. You can also purchase from Helios Pharmacy online - they also give excellent advice and this is where I buy mine.

You can buy tablets or pellets. Pellets are tiny so you are getting much more for your money!

Please remember that all medicine has contra-indications and may react with your prescribed medicine or with an existing condition that you may have. If in doubt, please check with your doctor and then consult a qualified practitioner.

My experience

From all the therapies and treatments I have experienced, I received the quickest and the best results from homeopathy and I am a committed fan. However, I went to numerous homeopaths who never seemed able to prescribe the correct remedy as they were using the answers that I gave to certain questions to 'guess' what Homeopath type of person I was. Most homeopaths diagnose from their experience and asking lots of questions about you, including odd ones like do you like snakes (no!) or thunderstorms (no!) which seem to be totally irrelevant to you but not to the homeopath. Then they use this information to match you to the 'constitutional' type of the different remedies.

However, as there are thousands of remedies, this does mean that getting the right one can be difficult. Most homeopaths will tell you at the beginning that it is a case of trial and error. You can go to a homeopath who uses a Vega machine which links up to your thumb and gives percentage readings of how good the remedy would be for you but it doesn't ask questions like 'is there a better remedy for you?' or 'will this remedy make any difference to the symptoms?'.

So one day I sat with my homeopathic book and my dowser and within ten minutes I selected a remedy that enabled me to lose water and weight for the first time in five years – this was Helphar Sulphur which is a remedy I still take every day, just to be sure!

This is where muscle testing and dowsing really come into their own. You can be accurate when selecting the remedy and the dose and it eliminates any guess work. Although these techniques are not used widely by homeopaths, they could be used by you to either check the homeopath's recommendations or chose your own remedy.

Depending on the individual, I will suggest organ remedies (such as thyroid or pituitary) as well as the persons 'constitutional' remedy (ie the remedy that the person needs to treat them as a whole person) as a boost to the endocrine system. Then usually a person will have a weekly remedy as well.

DON'T BELIEVE WHAT YOU READ IN THE NEWSPAPERS ABOUT HOMEOPATHY – IT REALLY DOES WORK!

Remember that you must consult a qualified practitioner or use some form of diagnostic tool to ascertain the remedy, the strength and for how long you should take the remedy. All products can have side effects so do your research before you take any remedies and make sure that they don't clash with any prescription medication that you have from your GP.

Potency is a hot subject when talking about homeopathy and there are many types of homeopaths who prescribe using totally different doses, some in liquid form and some in tablet form. You will see the remedies represented as a number and a letter, such as 6c or 200c. Many of the remedies that you buy over the counter will be in this range. However, my prescribing for conditions that are serious start with a remedy that is 200c. This progresses to 1M and can even go to 10M. However, Sarcodes (organ therapy) are always prescribed as 6-200c.

As this explanation is very brief, please surf the internet if you want to know more about homeopathy, as it contains a wealth of knowledge. I would also suggest that you buy a good homeopathic book for you to learn about the remedies, doses and how they work. I would suggest to begin with a book with pictures of the constitutional types. All the constitutional symptoms, likes and dislikes are normally listed for easy reference. You will soon be able to recognise certain types just from their picture. It really is fascinating.

How quickly do homeopathic remedies work?

If the problem is something like an upset tummy the results are very quick and you will notice a difference almost immediately. If the remedy is for arthritis or a more serious issue it may take up to a month for you to notice a difference as the remedy is 'healing' and not just 'masking' the problem. They will always heal the external problems first and work inwards (ie skin first and then joints) or they will heal the last issue to show itself first and then work backwards. Please persevere, as the results are well worthwhile.

How are homeopathic remedies taken?

Remedies can be administered by either:
1   Dropping the pellets under the tongue
2   Dissolving them in a small amount of water and drink
3   Grinding into a powder that is poured into the mouth

Please note the following:

1   Do not handle the pellets as they can easily be neutralized
2   Do not take a remedy thirty minutes before or after cleaning your teeth or drinking coffee as peppermint and coffee will neutralize the effects
3   Always tell your doctor that you are taking a homeopathy remedy

Listed below are the homeopathic remedies I recommend for appetite suppressants, weight and water loss. There are a lot more remedies available, but I have selected the ones I particularly like. Also your own constitutional remedy, that won't be listed below, might include the answer to your weight or water problem so don't restrict yourself just to the given list.

Weight loss recommendations:

I have listed homeopathy used to suppress your appetite in the chapter on appetite suppressants, as most of the prepared supplements on the market are mainly to do with appetite.

The remedies are listed in alphabetical order but I have marked the ones that I really recommend with an '*'. I have kept the explanations brief and to the point – you know where to go if you want to find out more information about them!

Antimonium crud
This remedy is for excess hunger even after eating

Calotropis Gigantea ***
This is used to reduce the fat without decreasing the weight in this way your flesh will be decreased, the muscles will become harder and firmer.

*Calcarea Carb**
For the person with a sluggish metabolism, fatigue, excess hunger and soft muscles. This person gains weight easily and has oedema

Capsicum
Good for obesity problems especially when you don't want to take exercise because you tire easily

Chelidonium
For liver support and improved fat metabolism

Fucas (from seaweed)*
For thyroid support. All seaweed products are excellent for the thyroid

Hydrocotyle Asiatica
This is another name for Gotu which is excellent for the circulatory system

Graphites*
For the large bone person with a large appetite who gains weight easily. This person has hunger both during meals and in-between meals.

Hephar Sulphur*
This remedy is for a flabby person with weak muscles. I have had excellent results with this remedy. It gave me very slim ankles and theys didn't swell up when I was flying. I take this remedy all the time.

Iodium (from iodine)*
For thyroid support and as an appetite suppressant. Also lessens water retention. The thyroid is normally short of iodine and needs additional supplies

Kali Carb
This remedy is generally used for older people with an obesity problem, who have puffy eyes and retain a lot of water

Lycopodium
Is an excellent remedy for liver weakness. Lycopodium often helps with indigestion, gas, bloating and constipation. Lycopodium helps with the too full feeling after eating

Natrum Carb
Stimulates cellular activity and increases oxidation and metabolism

Natrum Mur
Important remedy for thyroid and kidneys. (I have read a review which says 'bashful' kidneys – what a wonderful phrase!)

Natrum Sulphur
Liver support and improved fat metabolism

Nux Vomica
This is a good remedy for the person who overeats

Paullina Sol
Is homeopathic Guarana for stamina without any caffeine

Pulsatilla*
For feeling more hungry even after eating, improves indigestion from fatty foods. Supports metabolism and is great for weight loss

Spongia Tosta*
Is made from roasted sponge from the sea. Sponge contains significant amounts of iodine and bromine and are used both allopathically and homeopathically to treat goitre and other thyroid problems

St Johns Wort (Hypericum)*
Good for Seasonal Affective Disorder and weight loss. Excellent for the Pineal – remember not to go out into the sun when you are taking this remedy as it might make you hypersensitive

Staphysagria
This remedy is to be used if your weight could be caused by protection against violent people or if you have deep unresolved anger

Sulphur*
To ease cravings for carbs and sweets, help with morning appetite

Thuja
Good for people who are obese and have an excess of flabby tissues on the body. This remedy is also excellent for the skin tags that are caused by a thyroid problem and they disappear, like magic, in a couple of days.

Thyroidium
This is good for the thyroid gland and goitre conditions

Water retention remedies

Apis Mel*
This remedy is absolutely brilliant for getting rid of excess water

Berberis Vulgaris
A good remedy to support the bladder and the kidneys

Cantharis
Excellent support for the bladder and kidneys

Uva Ursi
Excellent support for kidneys

Organ therapy or sarcodes

Sarcodes is homeopathy prepared from the secretions or healthy tissues, including the endocrine glands, which are then dried. Typically these are ground and diluted as per homeopathic procedures.

These are normally tissues from calves and although I am totally against using anything from animals, I have found them to be of great use to me in my recovery. Before taking the tablet I now offer thanks to the animal that has allowed me to get better.

I use sarcodes all the time to target and activate the endocrine system. Sarcodes are always named after the organ that they originate from and a list of the sarcodes I use are listed below:

- Adrenals which is further split into cortex and medulla
- Gallbladder
- Hypothalamus
- Liver
- Pancreas
- Pineal
- Pituitary (whole) which is further split into anterior and posterior
- Serotonin
- Thyroid
- Thyroid-simulating hormone
- Thyroxin

Sarcode supplements

I debated whether to put these in the homeopathy or the herb section under supplements, but decided as we had just discussed sarcodes this would be the better option.

You can buy sarcodes as supplements, rather than in a homeopathic form. I do use these quite a lot and purchase them from a company called Nutri. As homeopathy works slowly, I use these as a boost to begin with at the beginning of a treatment.

Nutri sell a selection of the sarcodes shown in the homeopathy section. Nutri only sell through qualified therapists so you will have to contact them to find somebody in your local area.

Cells salts (also called tissue salts)

Cell salts are a set of twelve mineral salts created by a German homeopath, W.H.Schuessler, in the late 19th century. Although produced homeopathically, they were originally meant to be used as agents to restore the body's biochemical balance. They are produced in a low potency (3c or 6C) and can be purchased in your local health food shop. These are excellent to add to your supplements, especially if you are lacking iron or feeling run down.

Cell salts are so important because minerals are the foundation for enzyme activity in the body and serve as catalysts in energy cycles and functions. For example, the body must first have minerals to make vitamins or make use of vitamins regardless of the source. Cell Salts are used in the basic functioning of the cells including water balance, digestion, removing toxins, elasticity of the cells, oxygenation, nutrition, sodium/potassium balance etc

When I first treat a client, I will normally recommend that they take cell salts to boost their systems. The cells salts are:
- 3 Calcium minerals: calcium fluoride, calcium phosphate & calcium sulphate
- 3 Potassium minerals: kali mur, kali phosphate & kali sulphur
- 3 Sodium minerals: natrum phosphate, natrum sulphur & natrum mur
- Plus: ferrum phosphate (iron); magnesia phosphate (magnesium); ssilicea (silica)

There is an excellent remedy called Bioplasma from Elixirs.com which contains all twelve cell salts which I take every day, especially as I have severe problems with water retention and water seeping between my tissues. Elixirs also have lots more interesting information on their website about cell salts and how you can recognise when you have a deficiency.

Chapter 18:
HERBAL MEDICINE FOR WEIGHT LOSS

Herbal medicine is used to assist the body in its own instinctive attempts to self-heal. Herbs and other plant medicines have been used since the Stone Age, becoming more popular in the last decade as an alternative to standard medicine.

Herbalists use the leaves, flowers, stems, berries and roots of plants to prevent, treat and relieve illness. For instance, digitalis is used as a heart regulator and St John's Wort is a popular remedy for mild to medium depression and weight loss.

I use herbs with my clients mainly for boosting metabolism and cleansing and balancing the body's organs. Herbs really come into their own for cleansing the system. This is so important for detoxification and weight loss and then for eliminating toxins and keeping weight off and the metabolism boosted. For example cleansing the liver, kidneys and colon is essential for eliminating all old toxins and improving organ function. This in turn boosts well-being and weight loss. However, herbs have become increasingly popular in 'slimming pills' or 'appetite suppressants' so I have listed the most common ones that appear in these prepared supplements.
I have to confess that I don't prepare my herbs from scratch but I buy tinctures from Neal's Yard already made up which makes them so easy to take and absorb. Please buy the best herbs you can afford as not all manufacturers are equal.

One of my finds is black walnut which not only gets rid of parasites but boosts the metabolism as well. The majority of herbalists now recommend a brand of pre-made remedies and you can buy your own products in a health food shop.

I have listed my favourite herbs – the ones marked with an asterisk should be taken by everybody. You will notice that some of the names are familiar, such as St John's Wort and fucus, and we have talked about them already in the homeopathic chapter. As the plants are used both by herbalists and homeopaths there is a considerable amount of cross over but it is the preparation of them that differs. I don't talk a lot about

Chinese herbs as I don't have much experience of them – the only experience being of boiling up roots and drinking a revolting tea. Chinese medicine, however, is very successful so if your intuition leads you to it go to a registered Chinese medicine practitioner and get the remedies already made up, otherwise you could be drinking revolting tea as well!

I have listed appetite suppressants in a separate chapter, as most of the prepared supplements on the market are mainly to do with appetite.

Flower remedies

As well as herbs, later in this chapter I have listed the flower remedies that I have found to be useful in my quest for health. I have talked about Bach and Australian Flower remedies but haven't even touched on any other types, of which there are many. If you are drawn to flower essences do your research on the internet and use your intuition to choose which one you need.

Flower remedies are prepared by imprinting a flower's unique vibrational healing signature onto a carrier solution of brandy and water. This is achieved by working with flowers that are growing in the wild in an environment free from pollution. These flowers are placed in a bowl of pure water and left in direct sunlight for several hours. The flowers are then removed from the bowl and the remaining flower water is added to an equal amount of brandy, which acts as a preservative.

Selection of herbs – get your dowser out now!

Below I list a variety of herbs in alphabetical order. These herbs are for all the possible reasons you can't lose weight – be it for the thyroid, digestion, liver, hormones or water retention. Whatever your problem, you will find a herb here!

Angelica archangelica	It regulates the appetite and boosts the metabolism of the liver. It contains chrome, a mineral helping to regulate sugar metabolism, reducing sugar cravings and thus protecting against diabetes. On the emotional side it symbolises our guardian angel and we need our angels' support in weight loss diets as in

all other situations in life when we feel alone confronted with problems.

Ashwaganda	This is an Indian herb that is a major antioxidant and is used for stress. It also supports the immune system. As it reduces cortisol it is good for weight loss and hair growth. It can be good for the thyroid.
Avena sativa	Avena sativa is derived from the wild oat plant and is a well known restorative and nerve tonic, used to treat depression, low libido and lack of energy, as well as hypothyroidism. More recently it has also been shown to be effective in reducing high cholesterol levels.
Azadirachta indica	This is one of the best plants in Ayurvedic medicine and a good all-rounder.
Margosa tree, Indian lilac neem	Mostly helpful in cases of old or chronic disorders; it provides long term cleaning up, thus assisting the detoxification process and regulating the acid-base equilibrium
Banaba leaf extract	Banaba is a medicinal plant that grows in India, Southeast Asia and the Philippines. Traditional uses include brewing tea from the leaves as a treatment for diabetes and hyperglycaemia (elevated blood sugar). Also controls appetite and food cravings.
Betula alba , European birch	This is a diuretic; it also detoxifies the lymphatic system and purifies blood, which is most helpful during dieting, as the clear lymph fluid which circulates through our tissues to cleanse them is of the utmost importance in eliminating waste – liver health being a key to lymphatic health as the liver produces the majority of lymph. Betula works in synergy with the plants for liver – taraxacum and carduus.

Bitter melon*	Bitter Melon is used for reducing blood sugar and diabetes.
Bioperine®/ black pepper*	Bioperine® is an extract obtained from the black pepper fruit that is cultivated in the damp, nutrient-rich soil regions of southern India . The extract of piperine, called Bioperine® in the patented form, has been clinically tested in the United States. Bioperine® significantly enhances the bioavailability of various supplement nutrients through increased absorption.

The metabolic process that generates energy at the cellular level in the human body is called thermogenesis. Thermogenesis has been identified as a key factor in losing weight and then maintaining the weight loss.

Black walnut***	Black Walnut is an excellent metabolism booster and eliminates parasites that could be causing weight and/or water retention. It is also a kidney tonic and cures constipation. An excellent all round herb.
Bonsal	Bonsal comes from shellfish and is supposed to reduce body fat deposits in the belly, thighs and buttocks. It also makes sure that the fat from your last meal leaves your body before being digested.

I am going to try this one as soon as I can start taking supplements again.

Boldo leaf	Boldo Leaf is a native South American herb for the treatment of liver, gallbladder, and urinary problems.. It has been found to be a liver and gallbladder stimulant, as well as having antioxidant, diuretic, sedative, and anti-inflammatory properties.

Butternut	Butternut is good not only as a laxative, but also as a support treatment for various liver disorders so it is a good eliminator.
Carduus marianus St. Mary's Thistle (also known as Milk Thistle)****	Milk Thistle is a plant for the liver, protecting intact liver cells by preventing the entry of toxic substances. Also stimulates protein synthesis and thereby accelerates the regeneration process of liver cells. Everybody should take this remedy, especially if they drink alcohol!
Caralluma Fimbriata****	This plant is recommended by Dr Perricone in his book *Seven Secrets*. CF has been used in Indian medicine for centuries. It is a cacti that grows wild all over India and is eaten either as a cooked vegetable, in chutney or raw. Indians chew chunks of CF to suppress their appetite when they are away all day hunting. CF increases energy along with fat loss and can reduce your waist circumstance dramatically. CF not only inhibits fat synthesis but also increases the burning of fat – I am off to order some now!
Capsaicin	Food scientists in Taiwan report that Capsaicin – the natural compound that gives red pepper its spicy kick – can reduce the growth of fat cells. Use it in stir fries and put more than you usually would in your salads.
Cayenne	Cayenne pepper is thought to increase the metabolic rate – it's worth a try!
Cha de Burge	Cha de Burge (also called Café do mato in its native Brazil) is found in the forests of Brazil where it has long been used as a weight loss product and appetite suppressant. It is also used as a heart tonic and circulatory stimulant

which may help prevent or reduce fatty deposits and cellulite

Cinnamon

Recent studies have determined that consuming as little as one-half teaspoon of cinnamon each day may reduce blood sugar, cholesterol, and triglyceride levels by as much as 20%. Good for fat on the tummy. As it is a stimulant, it could raise the metabolic rate.

Citrus Aurantium Extract (bitter orange)*

Bitter Orange is used to increase the body's metabolic rate. It is also being investigated for it appetite suppressant functions – I have used this with some success.

Cleavers*

This herb is excellent for the urinary and lymphatic systems and should be used for detoxing. A must in everybody's cupboard.

Coleus forskohlii

Coleus forskohlii is a well-respected and often difficult to obtain Ayurvedic (Indian) remedy, traditionally used to treat high blood pressure. It also acts to stimulate the thyroid to release thyroid hormones and is therefore beneficial in the treatment of hypothyroidism.

Damiana

Damiana stimulates the circulation and promotes weight loss. It is also used as an aphrodisiac, so you have been warned!

Drosera rotundifolia sundew***

Although originally this plant was used for soothing coughs, it also helps people resist food cravings and goes into the depth of fat cells to eliminate excess stored fat – sounds good to me!

Fucus vesiculosis (kelp) **

Fucus vesiculosis, also called bladderwrack or kelp, is a sea vegetable which is a prime source of iodine - crucial in preventing thyroid problems. It has been used medicinally for thousands of years, especially in traditional

Chinese medicine. Apart from its beneficial effect on thyroid functioning, it is also used as a metabolic stimulant and can be found in many slimming remedies. A must if you have a thyroid problem.

Galium
A plant for digestion, it also has sedative properties and soothes nerves. People dieting often feel tense due to the frustration of not being able to eat as much as before.

Garcinia Cambogia****
Garcinia Cambogia is an extract of the Indian Brindall berry that has been found to dramatically increase the body's ability to convert food into glycogen. Glycogen is the body's fuel for energy consuming activities. When you have lots of glycogen in your body it triggers a signal to the brain telling it to suppress your appetite. The result is a marked decrease in the craving for fattening foods. In addition it slows the production of fat. This results in your cells burning it for energy at a faster rate. Not only do you eat less fat, but you also burn it faster. This sounds good to me!

Ginkgo
This is a plant for the mind and in this combination it supports the will to follow the diet successfully. Ginkgo also brings a good mood and serenity. This essence supports the liver functions and has antioxidant properties. Both properties are important in case of calorie restriction.

Guaraná****
Guaraná is a creeping shrub native to the Amazon Guarana acts as a general tonic and a mild stimulant and therefore it increases energy output. Guaraná increases the metabolic rate so it is good to be used as part of a weight-loss regimen. Guarana contains a compound almost identical to caffeine.

NOTE: Guarana is not recommended for those with high blood pressure or heart conditions.

Guggul***　　This Indian herb is used to lower cholesterol, boost the thyroid and combat Diabetes II. Great for weight loss.

Gymnema Sylvestre – the Sugar destroyer　　The main focus of Gymnema research is for blood sugar regulation and glucose metabolism. Don't know why they are researching because it has been used for this for 2,000 years!

Hibiscus Extract　　This can be drunk as a tea or taken as an extract. Hibiscus reduces obesity, shrinks a fat stomach and repairs a fatty liver. It also has anti cancer drugs and is good for kidney stones

Hoodia*****　　This seems to be by far the most important and effective appetite suppressant around and is widely sold in various guises. I have tried this myself with amazing effects so I would highly recommend you try this if you need to suppress your appetite at any time.

The Hoodia Gordonii plant is a herb, which grows naturally in the harsh desert conditions of the Kalahari desert of Southern Africa. For many generations the nomadic SAN tribe's people of the region have used the Hoodia Gordonii plant to suppress appetite and thirst during long hunting trips of several days duration

Although there are over twenty species in the Hoodia family, only the Hoodia Gordonii plant contains a natural appetite suppressant.

Irvingia Gabonensis*****　　This is also known by the common names wild mango, African mango, or bush mango and is in Al Sear's *Primal Lean Formula*. It is the latest thing for weight loss and is said to improve leptin levels which mean that you are not hungry and the fat is released from the cells. A must for anybody wanting to lose weight!

Juniper Berries

Used as a support for the kidneys and bladder so is therefore good for water retention Also combats Diabetes I and II.

Liquorice root

Liquorice root contains the chemical compound glycyrrhizin, which helps to stabilise the adrenal cortex hormone aldosterone. Aldosterone is responsible for regulating the fluids in your body. An excellent all-rounder for the adrenal glands but not to be taken if you have heart problems or high blood pressure.

Maca***

Maca grows in the Peruvian Andes and is one of the best remedies around for the menopause. It stimulates the pituitary and is therefore good for hormonal water retention and weight gain. A must for anybody who is peri- or menopausal.

Modifilan®

This is a potent seaweed extract harvested from pristine Arctic waters off the coast of Iceland, which has been shown to stimulate increased leptin production in fat cells by up to 18% through its ability to stimulate Thyroid Stimulating Hormone (TSH) in the adrenals. Stimulation of TSH in turn stimulates the production of leptin in fat cells.

Nelumbo nucifera (sacred lotus)***

This is Bali's slimming secret and may hold the key to helping you lose weight. Researchers were able to see this at work in a recent study. They found that sacred lotus appears to slow the natural process of making new fat cells and signals for the breakdown of existing fat at the same time. This tests very well and I have used it myself and would highly recommend it! This is in Al Sear's *Bali slim.*

Okoubaka aubrevillel

Okoubaka aubrevillel is an African root, it is the detoxifying plant, a major remedy for the 21st Century human being, who, in developed societies has unhealthy eating and living habits (fast food, excess consumption of alcohol).

Panax notoginseng

This is a well-known and commonly used traditional Chinese herb called 'Shan Qi' by master herbalists and was recently shown to also have unique metabolic properties, including naturally suppressing appetite and increasing leptin sensitivity.

PinnoThin

PinnoThin is a natural ingredient, obtained from a special oriental pine tree nut that can help stimulate the release of a hunger-suppressing hormone, so there's less chance you'll feel hungry. Recent research conducted on PinnoThin reveals that within thirty minutes of taking this supplement, people had less desire to eat and when they did eat, they ate significantly smaller portions. I haven't taken this myself but the reports and the results look good.

Slippery Elm

This is a great herb for digestion, but recent articles have shown that if you take 2 supplements before food, it gives you a quicker transit and you don't absorb so many calories

Stevia***

This is the best herb ever and should be in everybody's cupboard. It is a South American herb that is used if you need to sweeten anything. It also controls appetite and it excellent for controlling blood sugar. It really is the answer to our 'sweet' prayers!

Taraxacum officinale Dandelion***

Dandelion strengthens the liver detoxifying functions, helps the digestion process by stimulating bile production and fortifies the pancreas, spleen and stomach. It also has a mild laxative and diuretic effect and drains the lymphatic system – a good all-rounder!

Turmeric (also called curcumin)*****

There are many health benefits of turmeric, including weight loss. These benefits also come from curcumin, which is an ingredient in turmeric. This also provides turmeric with curcuminoids, which are believed to have health properties such as antioxidant, antibacterial and anti-inflammatory qualities. A good excuse to eat curry and add this to all types of foods such as soups, rice, eggs for the benefit every day. However, turmeric can stain your teeth as it is bright yellow, so you may want to take tablets!

White bean extract

White bean extract (cannellini beans) is now being used as an appetite suppressant and is a great weight loss supplement. You can either take the supplement or eat the beans, but my research shows that the supplement is better for weight loss. Several of my friends have had great success with this supplement and I now take it. It also balances your blood sugar levels.

Yerba Mate

Added to some appetite suppressants as it contains a substance similar to caffeine and is also an appetite suppressant. It is said to aid fatigue and is compared to green tea for its health benefits.

Yohimbe

Because it stimulates the central nervous system, it has been used to treat narcolepsy and for weight loss. Yohimbe increases fatty acid mobilisation, decreasing fat synthesis, which means it not only aids in weight loss, but actual fat reduction. Yohimbe is popular with bodybuilders. By stimulating the production of testosterone, it can help build muscle mass.

Other Herbs to include in your diet daily
I haven't listed all the herbs that you should be taking every day like coriander, garlic and ginger as this chapter would end up at twenty pages long!! All herbs have benefits and are potentially good for you, so experiment with them and add them to your cooking daily – I especially like eating the herb salads that are available now.

Herbs not to use
Research has shown that the following herbs can cause some problems so should be avoided. These herbs are sometimes part of a pre-packaged weight loss programme or in Chinese medicine so please look out for them on the labels:
- Ephedra
- Ephedrine
- Ma huan (ephedra)
- Sida cordifolia (ephedra)

Grasses

Green food is a popular term used to describe young grasses such as barley and wheat before they are converted into grain. The most nutritious part lies in the young green blades. These can be bought as supplements or in a drink – you don't have to chew on green blades! These really should form part of your daily routine.

They have the following benefits:
- Enhanced metabolism
- Anti–inflammatory
- Anti-oxidant
- Detoxification
- Includes numerous vitamins and minerals
- Makes your system alkaline

Sprouting

It is a very good idea to learn how to grow sprouts from seed. This is a very healthy form of eating and very easy and cheap to do.

Bach Flower Remedies

In the 1930s, Edward Bach developed thirty eight different remedies that have become known as Bach Flower Remedies. Through his work he found that flowers healed on a physical level and an emotional level as well and that both were related.

Bach Flower Remedies can be purchased from all health food stores and are available in either a tincture (which is preserved in brandy) or you can buy a tablet from a specialised outlet but these are more difficult to get. A must in everybody's bathroom cupboard is 'Rescue Remedy' which you take at any time that you are in a stressful situation or have had a shock. It is also extremely good for both children and animals.

Bach Flower Remedies do not have a specific weight loss remedy as they work quite similarly to homeopathy by having a 'constitutional' type. Buy a book or surf the Bach site on the net and select which flower remedy matches your personality type. This flower remedy will then help sort out your emotions and will in turn help curb your appetite and help you to lose weight. Crab Apple is very good for cleaning out and detoxing.

Australian Bush Flower Remedies

After the success that Dr Bach had with his flower remedies, many countries round the world prepared their own flower remedies from their own vast array of flowers and plants. One of the most popular after Bach Flower Remedies is the Australian ones. I list only a few as they are the ones with which I have had the most experience.

Old man banksia   An excellent remedy for low thyroid function – I have used it with great success

Bush fuscia   This is the remedy for kick starting the hypothalamus

261

Bush iris   This is the best remedy for the pineal and the lymphatic system

Yellow cowslip orchard   This is the remedy to get all parts of the pituitary working in harmony together

Teas

Teas can also help with weight loss – but not with milk and sugar!

Green tea   Green tea has come to prominence in the west over the past few years mainly due to the benefits that can be derived from drinking it. Green tea contains more vitamins than black tea and is also a wonderful source of antioxidants. These antioxidants have been proven essential for the body to maintain a healthy balance

Loose teas: Pu erh   This tea has the ability to assist in weight management. This type of tea is widely drunk in China with meals to aid digestion. Its ability to increase digestion of fatty foods with incredible efficiency is why it is recommended that this tea is drunk with meals. It is also proven to reduce cholesterol levels when drunk regularly, again with meals – apparently when it was announced that Victoria Beckham drank this, the shop sold out within hours!

Oolong tea   This is a new one I have found that is once again the 'latest thing'! Supposedly cuts appetite and increases the metabolism and is vouched for by Ophrah!

Other interesting herbs

While I am writing this book, it seems sensible to write about other herbs that I have found to be useful along the way. The two I want to add here are Oil of Black Pepper and Oil of Basil as they have tremendous properties.

Oil of Black Pepper   Apparently, Oil of Black Pepper has been used for thousands of years as a 'cure all' but is particularly good for the immune system. We all take this oil including my dogs!

Oil of Oregano   This is recommended by Dr Perricone in his book *Seven Secrets* as a potent antibiotic and a powerful radical fighter. My dog Milie took this oil as she had a recurring nose infection due to an allergy to grass.

Chapter 19:
EVERY OTHER NUTRIENT YOU WILL NEED FOR WEIGHT LOSS

Because the nutrients in our food are so bad and everybody absorbs vitamins and minerals in a different way, it is important to ensure that you take daily supplements of the additional nutrients you need. When you read the very informative book, *The Human Time Bomb, The Slow Poisoning of America'* or you listen to Al Sears and Joe Mercola, you will see that because of poor soil quality, pesticides and the age of the food, there are very little nutrients left for you to absorb. We talk about having five fruit and vegetables a day but actually these days nearer eight would be the required amount and this could become difficult to eat every day.

'How do you know which ones you need, how often and what dose?' is a question I am often asked. Well, by now I am surprised that you don't know that answer. Get a really good book on vitamins and minerals and get your dowser out or start muscle testing. Use your intuition as well – do you think you may not need a mineral but fancy the sound of it? Dowse to see if it is good for you at the moment. Please remember that you must dowse for what dosage you need daily, when to take that dosage and for how long you need take these supplements. Some may be forever but some may be on a short term basis only. These nutrients should be backed up by other nutrients that are contained in the other chapters and are relevant to that particular problem. The list here is only a very basic one.

You will need to invest in a good book because vitamins and minerals etc need to be taken at different times of the day and sometimes not together – so you need more help with this than that you will be getting in this section. I don't plan to explain each supplement as there is already of wealth of information out there.

It is important for exhausted dieters to take their supplements and most probably you will need quite high doses to begin with so don't be surprised!

I would love you to get everything that you need from your food but to begin with this will most probably be unrealistic, especially if you have a thyroid problem or have been dieting for a long time. Please do not listen to the reports in the newspapers that say that vitamin supplements are a waste of time and money, because they are not! On the other hand, don't think that after a couple of weeks you will have absorbed all you need and that won't require them anymore. You need to take supplements for at least three months before you see any difference and especially when taking things like Omega 3 or other fish oils – you will be taking those for life.

People that have been dieting for a long time can also be malnourished. You are cutting calories and perhaps not getting all the nutrients you need. This was my problem my entire life as I have been living on less than 800 calories a day, most of which were carbohydrates to keep me full, so I was getting very few nutrients.

Vitamins

To be quite frank, you will need to supplement your diet with all vitamins to begin with, to become and to remain healthy. Using your newly purchased book on vitamins and minerals, you will be studying what foods you need every day to incorporate these vitamins into your daily diet.

However, in my opinion, the most important vitamins for losing weight are listed below:

Vitamin A:
This works with Zinc and Vitamin E to manufacture thyroid hormones. It is needed for all sorts of functions, including healthy night vision.

All the B vitamins *including B1, B2, B3, B6, Folic Acid (B9), Pantothenic Acid (B5), B12, Inositol and Paba:*
These are important vitamins in terms of weight loss and they are often known as the 'stress' vitamins. Vitamins B3 and B6 are especially important because they help to supply fuel to cells, which are then able to burn energy. Vitamin B6 together with zinc is necessary for the production of pancreatic enzymes which help you to digest food. If your digestion is good, you will be much more likely to use your food efficiently, instead of storing it as fat!

Vitamins B2, B3 and B6 are necessary for normal thyroid hormone function production, so any deficiencies in these can affect thyroid function and consequently affect metabolism. B3 is also a component of the glucose tolerance factor which is released every time your blood sugar rises. Vitamin B5 is involved in energy production and helps to control fat metabolism. Without Vitamin B12 your body cannot metabolise cholesterol.

Vitamin C:
Needed for absorption of nutrients. Dr Perricone's research has shown that Vitamin C can improve the body's ability to oxidize fat and also reduce fatigue.

Vitamin D:
Take as a supplement. Can also be topped up by the oil that you take in your fish oil and is good for every metabolic process – a must for everybody to take everyday for the rest of their lives. D3 is the best type to take and it must be combined with vitamin K to receive the full benefits. Now shown to release leptin which signals to the brain that the stomach is full and is good for releasing stomach fat as well! Remember to have fifteen minutes a day in sunlight without protection (not mid-day, obviously!) so you can get your Vitamin D this way as well. Please take K2 at the same time as this helps with absorption.

Vitamin E:
This helps absorb fat correctly and works with Vitamin A and Zinc to manufacture thyroid hormones.

Antioxidants:
Antioxidants are involved in the prevention of cellular damage - the common pathway for inflammation, cancer, ageing and a variety of diseases. Antioxidants are normally referred to as vit C, vit E and beta-carotene (which is the precursor of vitamin A) but minerals and enzymes can also help counteract this cellular damage.

Coenzyme 10:
CoQ10 is a powerful natural antioxidant that also plays a key role in converting the food we eat into metabolic energy. For weight loss, a study showed that people on a low-fat diet doubled their weight loss when taking CoQ10 compared to those using diet alone. It helps the body to release fat and use it for energy. Al Sears does an excellent

quality supplement which is better than supplements available in health food shops.

Minerals

Zinc:
This is an important mineral in appetite control and a deficiency can cause a loss of taste and smell, creating a need for stronger tasting foods (which tend to be sweeter, saltier and more fattening!) Zinc also functions with vitamins A and E to manufacture the thyroid hormones. Also improves your sex life!

Magnesium:
This is needed for a better metabolism and better digestion. Also excellent for PMS and menopause systems, so could help alleviate hormonal water retention.

Selenium:
Selenium deficiency can affect metabolism of thyroid hormones and is therefore essential for weight loss.

Calcium:
You might not think that calcium is important in weight loss and metabolism. However, recent clinical studies demonstrate a positive relationship between calcium intake and weight loss and can reduce the risk of being overweight by as much as 70%.

Manganese:
Manganese helps regulate fat metabolism and blood-glucose. It is needed for a healthy thyroid function which itself is essential to maintain a healthy weight.

Chromium Polynicotinate:
This mineral has been the most widely researched nutrient in relation to weight loss. Chromium is needed for the metabolism of sugar and without it insulin is less effective in controlling blood sugar levels and it totally stops you feeling hungry. This is a must for everybody who struggles to control their weight.

Al Sears has just found that Chromium Polynicotinate acts like HCA and helps turn on a number of genetic switches. It also turns off two genes that make brown fat, which is the hardest to shed. It powers down the gene that provides antioxidant support to your fat cells which means that it accelerates your fat cell death while the other types of cells survive – I really like the sound of this!

Chromium needs to be taken along with L'Carnitine otherwise the nutrients you are taking won't get into your cells.

Vanadium:
This helps regulate blood sugar so is good for appetite and controlling your weight.

Lecithin:
Lecithin forms a shield around your cells so that fat can't wriggle in and plump them out.

Iodine:
Essential for the thyroid. Kelp and spirulina are two good ways of ensuring that you have enough iodine for your thyroid. They are made out of seaweed which is full of iodine in a natural way.

Iron:
A friend of mine swears that if her iron levels get low her weight rockets. Iron is essential for body functions and giving you energy as well

Digestion

A healthy digestion will help with weight loss and then maintaining that loss for the rest of your life. Once again you will need help in the form of probiotics and enzymes to ensure that the food is broken down correctly and all the nutrients can be absorbed.

Probiotics:
Buy a supplement or have a daily drink of kefir (but remember to ask your body if you need it every day. Kefir has approximately 66 good bacteria whereas most capsules have about 14. You must take a capsule probiotic with your food to aid digestion and help eliminate constipation. A probiotic contains good bacteria such as acidophilus to keep your gut healthy and your digestion on top form. Over the years, because of diet and antibiotics, the bacteria in our gut can be seriously affected which causes a breakdown in the digestive process.

Enzymes:

Buy a supplement. There are seven basic types of digestive enzymes each with various sub-classifications and differing functions. The basic enzymes and their specific functions are as follows: amylase digests starches, cellulase digests fibres, lactase digests dairy products, lipases digest fats, oils and triglycerides, maltase digests starch and grains, proteases digest proteins and sucrase digests sugars.

Your body produces enzymes, which work to break down fats, proteins, sugars, carbohydrates, fibres, starches and lactose into small particles. Enzymes also work to release fibre-bound nutrients (nutrients that are 'stuck to fibre'), allowing minerals to be more available to your body.

So as well as a probiotic, it is essential to take a supplement containing all the digestive enzymes.

Other supplements to take

Lipoic acid:

Alpha Lipoic Acid is a powerful antioxidant which fights off the damaging effects of free radicals and also regenerates other antioxidants such as vitamin C, vitamin E and glutathione back to their active state. If it is combined with amino acids it is said to be one of the new answers to ageing!

Resversatol:

Talking about new wonder drugs, Resveratrol at this time is the in thing. It is obtained from red grapes and red wine but be warned you would have to drink 100 glasses a day for the benefits!

It is supposed to be anti-ageing, anti-cancer, anti-inflammatory and life-prolonging.

Now being hailed as a cure-all, scientific studies are showing that it may help you to lose weight and keep the weight off. French scientists have developed a drug called SRT1720 that is the chemical cousin of resveratrol that tricks the body into burning off fat even when on a high fat diet. You would have to drink gallons of wine to get the same affect! I take it.

Pycnolgenol:

Pycnolgenol is a natural plant extract originating from the bark of maritime pine trees and is known as a super strength antioxidant. Nicholas Perricone reports that Pycnogenol delays the uptake of glucose from a meal 190 times more than prescription medications, preventing the typical high glucose peak in the bloodstream after a meal. It also helps with Syndrome X because of the way it works with insulin and complex carbohydrates. I have used this for some time and it has helped my eyesight.

Super-Greens:
These are a mixture of all the vegetables and fruit that you will need on a daily basis and a scoop is added to a drink – so it is an easy and affective way to get the nutrition. These can be purchased from many suppliers so do your research on the internet and see which one jumps out at you.

Collagen:
As we get older our collagen fibres die and this is one of the reasons that our skin becomes old and wrinkly! If you are dieting and you want your skin to snap back, it is essential to add a collagen supplement to your diet. The improvement in your skin is amazing.

Al Sears and Joe Mercola – my favourite doctors!

I could go on for pages about other supplements that will help improve your health and help you lose weight. New important supplements are being discovered all the time, so what I am going to suggest you do is go to the websites of these two doctors and study their supplements and dowse or muscle test to see if you require them. I am not on commission by the way!

Chapter 20:
ESSENTIAL OILS AND WEIGHT LOSS

One book that should be in everybody's bookcase is a book on aromatherapy and essential oils. Essential oils are extracted from plants by various methods and have been used for thousands of years for their perfume and their healing properties.

Essential oils are made from plants that have undergone an extraction process. These plant extracts have been known for their therapeutic quality and have been used over thousands of years. When you buy essential oils, please buy the most expensive you can find that are also organic. In this case you really do get what you pay for.

Essential oils can be used in the following ways:
- Added to a carrier oil for massage
- Added to a burner or aroma diffuser
- Added to a bath
- Put directly on the skin as a healing method. (The only oils that should be put directly on the skin are lavender and tea tree oils.)

A book will list all of the applications of the various oils, along with any contraindications. These contraindications are very important, especially if you are pregnant. I will only be listing the oils that I think are good for weight loss but there are a myriad other uses and that is why you need to buy yourself a good book. If you have a baby, massage is simply the best way to bond with it. Essential oils can be used but before you start, I would suggest that you purchase a book specifically for essential oil massage for babies.

Please remember that anybody can have intolerance or an allergic reaction to any substance so before using any oil, do a small patch test to see if it suits you.

How to choose an essential oil

I mentioned in the paragraph above about purchasing a good book on oils, so you can study which oil is best used for which problem.

However, this is where your diagnostic tools come in extremely handy as you can use your crystal pendulum dowser or muscle testing to select the oil, or oils, that are best for you at that particular time for that particular issue. This really does take all the guess work out of trying to find the correct one. This is also essential if you are recommending it to somebody else or for a child. You can also try using your intuition and see which oil you think is best. Usually one will jump out from the page at you.

Aromatherapy massage

An aromatherapy massage is totally different from the normal massage. The aromatherapy massage is more of a lymph drainage massage, using a mixture of oils added to a carrier oil (for example, olive oil or nut oil). The therapist should not mix the oils before she has gone through your symptoms with you (ie the oils should not be premixed) as they should be totally matched to your requirements. The therapist should use a diagnostic tool, like dowsing or muscle testing, to select the oils and how many drops you need of it.

Sometimes the therapist will ask you to smell an oil to confirm that it is one you like – there is no point doing a massage with a smell that makes you feel sick or equivalent. It's like getting on an airplane having sprayed yourself with more than one perfume at Duty Free, only to smell the one you don't like for the rest of the flight!

However, If you really do not like the smell of the end mix of oils, you must tell the therapist, as this blend is not the correct one for you and it should be re-mixed.

The therapist will then add the selected oils to a bottle of massage oil, give it a good shake and apply it all over the body. The massage should last approximately 1 to 1 ½ hours. The therapist should also be able to adapt her routine to spend more time on areas of the body that need more work. For example, if you have a frozen shoulder, more time should be spent in this area.

If you find the type of massaging used during an aromatherapy massage is not what you like, perhaps it's not relaxing enough or not firm enough, again tell the therapist how you'd like it to be done.

Oil burners and incense sticks

Incense sticks are normally prepopulated with a perfume and your favourite can be on hand to burn at any time. I personally love incense sticks and have them burning in my house (and garden) at all times. Incense is used for cleansing

You can buy oil burners anywhere. I like the ones with a big bowl at the top as they don't burn dry too quickly. Place water in the bowl and add a few drops of an oil to the water. Light the tea light candle and once this heats up the water, the oil will start to burn, creating a wonderful perfume. A tip here is to keep tealights in the freezer and they will last longer than the normal three hours. Also if you were to burn a vanilla tea light you have the added benefit of an appetite suppressant as well!

Aroma diffusers

Essential oils are excellent for nose and congestion problems, ie eucalyptus and for relaxing, lavender and clary sage. It is not safe to go to sleep with an oil burner alight in the bedroom for obvious reasons but aroma diffusers are completely safe. They are electrically operated and when the water level in the reservoir reaches the lowest level, the diffuser switches itself off.

You can add drops of your favourite oils into your bath which is especially good for relaxation purposes. Don't pour oils into the bath under hot running water as this can destroy their effectiveness. I usually pour in the oils after I have run the bath and give them a quick swirl round.

Essential oils used directly on the skin

The only two essential oils that can be used directly on the skin are lavender and tea tree – it is very important that you remember this, as oils can be toxic if used in quantity. Lavender is used as a general healer for cuts and burns and is wonderful as a face or body lotion. Tea tree is more antiseptic and is used on spots and infections.

I have an entire book on uses for tea tree oil which include taking white marks off tables and lots of other uses that you wouldn't have guessed in a million years!

All other oils must be diluted in an appopriate liquid (for example, body lotion, hand cream, carrier oil or equivalent) before being added to the skin.

Essential oils which aid weight and water loss

Myrtus communis (Morocco)	This is an excellent oil to support the thyroid, increase the metabolism and balance the endocrine system.
Bladderwrack (focus)	Not used much as an essential oil these days as it is taken more as a herbal or homeopathic remedy. However, it is an excellent support for the thyroid so could be mixed with a carrier oil and put directly over the thyroid gland.
Hyssop	This oil regulates lipid metabolism.
Other oils that are good for weight loss	• Grapefruit • Lemon • Orange • Rosemary • Sandalwood • Frankincense

Essential oils which are good for the adrenals

Pine (Pinus sylvestris) and Spruce (Picea mariana)
These oils help revive your adrenal glands. Use this mixture in a massage oil or in your bath, which is excellent for adrenals:
- 4 drops pine (Pinus sylvestris)
- 2 drops spruce (Picea mariana)
- 2 drops lavender
- 1 ounce carrier oil

Essential oils which are good for releasing water retention (including kidneys and bladder)

- Benzoin (my favourite)
- Juniper
- Pettigrain
- Cedarwood
- Cypress
- Fennel

Essential oils which are good for suppressing the appetite

Patchouli

As discussed in the chapter on appetite suppressants, Patchouli is excellent for reducing the appetite and desire to eat

Other Appetite Suppressant Oils:

- Vanilla
- Lemon/Melissa
- Basil
- Oregano

Essential oils which are good for Cellulite

Use your intuition (or another diagnostic tool) and select approximately five of the following oils that will help improve your cellulite. Add those oils to a carrier oil and then massage daily over the area that has cellulite:

Grapefruit	Lemon	Orange	Rosemary
Geranium	Juniper	Lavender	Pine
Benzoin	Basil	Oregano	Sage

Essential oils which are good for women's problems

These are used for any period problems, the menopause and PMS and are very affective for hormonal water retention:

Clary sage	Cypress	Melissa	Pine
Geranium	Lemon	Chamomile	Rose Otto
Rosemary			

Essential oils which are good for the lymphatic system

These oils will stimulate the lymphatic system:

Sandalwood   Cypress   Lemon/Orange   Frankincense
Pettigrain

Essential oils which are good for the skin

These oils are beautiful for the skin and can be added to your normal face and body lotions. I particularly like Frankincense and when I apply it I can almost feel the wrinkles disappear!

- Rose Otto
- Lavender
- Sandalwood
- Frankincense

Other issues

I have just listed the oils I use for weight and water loss but there are many other issues that can also cause weight gain, such as digestion and constipation, which can be alleviated with oils, so I would suggest that you identify the essential oils you need for your particular problems.

Section 6

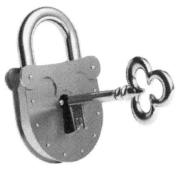

THERAPIES AND
TECHNIQUES
TO RELEASE WEIGHT

Chapter 21:
EMOTIONAL FREEDOM TECHNIQUE

There are a number of different meridian therapies, most of which are based on the ancient Chinese system of body meridians, which are also used during acupressure and acupuncture treatments. The one I am going to show you here is Emotional Freedom Technique, also known as EFT™.

When a person is calm and relaxed, the flow of energy through the meridian system is calm and steady. However emotional upsets of any kind – for instance unhappiness, stress, anger, trauma, fear, panic – affect the energy flow immediately; it becomes disturbed and distressed as our thoughts and emotions spiral off the calm centre state. In the early 1980s, Dr Roger Callahan found that instead of trying to control our thoughts or emotions mentally, the calm state of 'even flow' could more easily be restored by touching the meridian system, by gently tapping or holding the main meridian points. Once the meridian system has calmed, mind and body naturally follow suit and tranquility and balance are restored. He then developed his own technique called TFT.

These techniques are excellent for releasing the emotions that could be causing you to hold onto your weight and are equally as good in reinforcing healthy patterns of eating and getting rid of any cravings you may have. Hypnotherapists, counsellors and specialists in the medical profession are now using these techniques to speed up the rate of recovery. Clients who have been in therapy for years have had much quicker and more positive results, which is beneficial for both client and practitioner.

How EFT™ was started

Following on from Roger Callahan's discovery that his clients healed their issues much quicker when you touched or tapped on an acupuncture point, Gary Craig investigated this technique and took it to new levels. He called it Emotional Freedom Technique (EFT™ for short). EFT™ has been clinically effective in thousands of cases of trauma and abuse, panic and anxiety, fears and phobias, and cravings and addictions, as well as depression and weight problems for both humans and animals. EFT™ is a very simple technique where you tap lightly on certain meridian points whilst repeating a phrase and it can be done anywhere at any time. If it is inconvenient to tap the points, you can visualise tapping them and that will have the same affect. You can tap at any time, when watching the television, in the car or my favourite is on the toilet!

It is always a good idea to replace what you are healing with a positive statement so it is a good idea to write this down before you start so you know what you want to say. There has been masses amount of research and it has been proven that EFT™ can get to places in the brain and body to clear beliefs, trauma etc that other therapies can't.

In Appendix II is the précis of an EFT™ document that you can scan, then print and carry around with you for your convenience so you always know the points and the routines. There are many forms of EFT™ so the routines may differ when you look at other practioner's videos but don't worry as they are all doing the same good work! Some are easier than others. In my book called 'Unlock your maximum potential', I outline the 'long version' of the EFT routine, which includes humming, singing and eye movements – please stop laughing! It is highly affective and if you find that your issue or trauma isn't healing, then I suggest that you use the long version. For ease of use I have decided to use the shorter version in this book, but full details of the long version are given in Appendix II if you want to investigate it further.

When using EFT™, it is vital that you keep a record of whatever you are doing and your results and this way you can track your improvements. Also, this technique brings up deep emotions, feelings and old situations which need to be worked on. Therefore you need to carry your journal around and write down and investigate the memories that suddenly come to you.

Exciting new uses for EFT™

I was thinking about the problems with losing weight, mainly loose skin and the boobs heading south, so I thought why not use EFT™ on these? You could also use hypnosis (ask your hypnotherapist to devise a statement for you) and self-hypnosis. So why not tap on the problems that you think you might face or have already faced and see what difference it makes.

For example, if you wanted your boobs to be bigger or fuller there may be reasons that your subconscious doesn't want this to happen. Using the intensity number that we talk about in this section it will identify different aspects of the belief or the problem. If the problem is loose skin, it would be good to do an intensity reading and see if there are any beliefs that need changing, for example 'if I lose weight I will certainly get loose skin', or if there is anything else that stops your skin snapping back into place when your weight reduces, because it is only your belief that it won't happen. There is no reason why it can't happen – I cannot stress this enough. For these types of issues I would suggest that perseverance is the key and that you should tap on it every day.

So how could you use EFT™?
- Skin snapping back into place after weight loss
- Having a gastric band without an operation
- Boobs becoming firmer and perkier (you could try larger if you wanted!)
- Your skin becoming line free and tight along the jaw bone – you could try a face lift or looking 10 years younger
- Losing weight or becoming toned in a particular place that you haven't yet had much success with
- Tightening muscles without exercise (again this could be used for the face or specific areas)
- To improve your eyesight

How to use EFT™

Over the next few pages I am going to explain to you in depth how EFT™ works. It may seem very confusing but after a couple of rounds it will get easier and quicker. On **youtube** I have a video of me demonstrating all the points and how to tap, so I would suggest you follow this until you are completely confident. Remember, practice makes perfect!

Try it on everything for you and your children:
- Addictions and cravings
- Grief
- Weight problems
- Trauma
- Phobias

- Pain
- Depression
- Lack of memory and learning
- Allergies and intolerances
- STRESS
- Bullying

How to use EFT™ on you and your family

EFT™ is excellent for everybody and I would suggest that you use it for yourself and your family – especially your children. If you can find out from your children every day anything that has happened to them that is negative, such as a cruel put-down by a teacher or a pupil, they will be free of this 'baggage' later in life. If you are using EFT™ on your children or somebody else, follow the instructions for Surrogate Tapping in Appendix II or you can tap on your children or teach them how to do it for themselves.

It is a good idea to practice on yourself so you become familiar with the routines and the short cuts. Remember the more you use it the quicker the routines will become and you will have more confidence.

When the problem has been solved, it is a good idea to continue tapping on it for a couple of days to ensure that everything has been cleared 100% so that it doesn't return. These additional aspects are called 'Tailenders' which may be holding the problem in place.

Simple EFT™ Instructions

Using EFT™ may seem a little confusing and complicated to start with. However, after a couple of rounds you get more confident and quicker – I cannot stress this enough. When you are more experienced there are various shortcuts you can use. For example, the Set Up Statement is not always needed so you can cut this out. Sometimes just tapping on the facial points are enough to release what you are working on. This is easier and can be done quickly at any time. When you are very experienced your intuition will guide you to use only certain points. However, if you are stuck or the problem is not releasing you need to revert back to the whole EFT™ procedure. Even though I am only showing you the simple or shorter version, I show you all the points in the diagram as you may need them for a specific tapping routine.

EFT™ Tapping Points

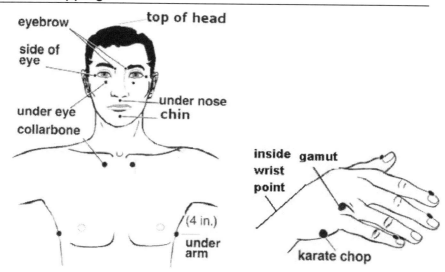

How to find the points

TOP = Top of the head
Right in the centre (as per the diagram) or you can lay your hand flat across the top

EB = Eyebrow
At the beginning of the eyebrow, above the nose

SE = Side of the Eye
At the end of the natural eyebrow arch, just where the temple commences

UE = Under the Eye
Under the eye on the bony part of the eye orbit (NOT the soft fleshy area under your eye)

UN = Under the Nose
Under the nose, just above the upper lip

CH = Chin
Centrally on the chin, in the crease

CB = Collar Bone

At the beginning of the collar bone, about 1inch (2.5cm) below the collarbone either side of the V part of your collarbone/throat area

UA = Under the Arm
Approximately one hand's width down from the armpit, on the side of the body. In ladies, about half way down where a bra strap would be, in men, level with the nipple, (normally feels tender)

TH = Thumb
On the outside nail bed corner of the thumbnail

IF = Index Finger
On the thumb-side of the nail bed of the index finger

MF = Middle Finger
On the thumb-side of the nail bed of the middle finger

LF = Little Finger
On the thumb-side of the nail bed of the little (baby/pinky) finger

KC = Karate Chop
On the side of the hand, level with fold of the palm of the hand, just under aninch (2.5cm) from the little finger joint

GP = Gamut point
On the back of the hand, approximately ½ inch (1.5cm) above and between the Little finger and ring finger knuckles

Take a few moments to touch and tap each point. Get to know these points. There may be different feelings at each point or there may be none at all. You may notice 'shifts' in feelings when you tap or touch these points or none at all. You may yawn a lot, sigh or cry – all of these reactions are totally normal and are signs that emotions are being released. You can tap on either side or you can tap on both sides at once. Usually you use two fingers but on the CB you can use all your fingers to cover a larger area.

Set Up Statements

I can understand that when you start, what to put in the Set Up Statement can be very confusing so I have given you plenty of examples below. I have also varied the endings (eg I deeply and utterly love and accept myself) so you can use other alternatives that may suit you better.

Contacting and getting in touch with the problem

In order to focus the tapping on the correct issue it is necessary to focus the mind on the problem by using a statement which represents the problem = how you are feeling about the problem eg: 'I crave crisps'. This is called creating the Set Up Statement.

- This Set Up Statement needs to be spoken aloud, with feeling, so that you're hearing and feeling yourself say the phrase
- The statement needs to ring true for you = you get feedback when you say it
- The statement is about YOUR PROBLEM therefore the words have to make sense to YOU and ONLY YOU
- The more frank and truthful you can be about your feelings, the more intense a change you will experience (you can swear if you want!)
- After formulating the Set Up Statement - and before starting tapping the KC point, simply say yourself: "Give me a number to show the intensity/discomfort of my feelings, 10 high and 1 or zero no feelings at all". The technical name for this intensity is Subjective Units of Distress/Discomfort or SUDS. The purpose of the exercise is for the number or the SUDS to be reduced to zero after a couple of rounds of EFT™.

Examples of Set Up Statement might be:
- I hate my job
- I crave crisps
- I hate my weight
- My shoulders are tense
- I am going to feel deprived if I diet
- I'll never be my goal weight
- I am hungry all the time/I am never full
- I have hidden issues that I don't want to look at
- I can't exercise and I don't have the time
- I am greedy
- I am not satisfied
- My family are fat so I will be fat too
- I have been called fat all my life so I live up to my name
- I have hormonal water retention
- I have severe oedema
- My thyroid doesn't function correctly

- Even though I can't let go/Even though I have this fear of letting go
- My metabolism only works at 70%
- My thyroid doesn't work properly
- I am on medication that slows my body down
- I don't have enough T3 in my bloodstream
- I have too much weight to lose
- If I am slim I will get too much attention and not feel safe
- I have been abused and use my weight as protection
- It is too hard and I will fail
- I hate myself/I am disgusted with myself

The Set Up

The Set Up consists of the following:
1. Stating 'Even though ...'
2. I deeply and completely love and accept myself (or words that are right for you)
3. Tap the KC Spot whilst saying this full phrase aloud – done three times in all

Using the first example of 'I have too much weight to lose' you would:
1. Tap on the KC spot saying out loud
2. "Even though I have too much weight to lose, I deeply and completely love and accept myself"
3. Do this three times

Whilst tapping the KC spot and repeating this phrase put as much emphasis as possible into the phrase when you are saying it. If you don't feel able to say "I deeply and completely love and accept myself" choose a similar phrase that is right for you.

The Sequence and Reminder Phrase

You now select a short form of your Set Up which could be:
- Fear of being attractive, Hate myself, I always fail, Too Hard

Following the Set Up it is now necessary to tap all the points, tapping them at least 7 times on each point, starting from the Eye Brow (EB) to Under Arm (UA) followed by Top of the Head (TOP) to end the sequence.

This is called the Sequence. As you tap each point, repeat a shortened version of the Set Up. This shortened version is called the Reminder Phrase.

Using the previous example:
"Even though I have too much weight to lose
I deeply and completely love and accept myself"

The Reminder Phrase (shortened version) would be: "Too much weight" and you would say this phrase whilst tapping on each point. You can shorten it even more simply to "weight".

The reason for repeating the Reminder Phrase is that the mind can become easily distracted and so by repeating this phrase you are focussing on that phrase which means you are connecting with the blocked/disturbed energy.

If you are doing multiple rounds of tapping, you only need to use the Set Up Statement once. After every few rounds take a new reading of the SUDS or intensity level and continue until it gets as low as possible. Change the Reminder Phrase if it feels appropriate. If you want to change the Set Up Statement or Reminder Phrase I would suggest that you go back to the start again and change the wording. Add anything new that might have shown itself during the tapping.

When the SUDS come down

You normally tap on the negative until the SUDS or intensity numbers comes down under 5. When this happens you can then add a positive affirmation at the end of the Set Up Statement:

Avoid at all costs using negative phrases such as:
"I will be slim and attractive"
"I will stop overeating"

Rephrase affirmations so that they are reframed in a positive light eg:
"I am a healthier person"
"I am slim and attractive"
"I eat healthily"

If this doesn't sit well with you try
"I am getting slimmer each day"

So the new Set Up would be:

"Even though I have too much weight to lose, I deeply and completely love and accept   myself" and I am getting slimmer each day"

Then you add 'Choices'

Pat Carrington, a very experienced EFTer is very fond of using choices within her set up statements. Also the word STILL sounds very innocuous but it means that your subconscious is still trying to hang onto the problem! So it is essential that it is cleared.

1. **First step – SUDS 10 to 5**
   Even though I don't want to lose weight I deeply and completely love and accept myself
2. **Second step – SUDS 5 to 1/2**
   Even though I **still** don't want to lose weight I deeply and completely love and accept myself
3. **Third step – SUDS 1/2 to 0**
   Even though I **still** don't want to lose weight I deeply and completely love and accept myself and **I now choose to lose weight and become the real me**

Personality parts of you and beliefs

Sometimes there are personality parts of you that don't want to let go of a particular problem and this could be another reason for a problem not clearing. These parts can be from a past life or this life and think they are still in the time frame where the trauma or the problem occurred. So by using EFT™ you need to identify who these parts are, what was the trauma and why are they hanging on for grim death!

I could not release the belief that I did not deserve to lose weight or become fit and healthy. I had been using all tools at my disposal for some time and, although the intensity would go down, then the next time I checked the intensity had risen again and this is because more issues were coming up to be cleared. So I had to work on all layers of the 'onion' of my 3 yr old self until all these beliefs were released and I then put in new positive beliefs in their place.

It is important that you work specifically with all these parts and ask if you have 100% of their cooperation because, until you get 100%, the problem or belief won't clear. Talk to them and explain that this is now and things are very different – that you are safe, free or whatever the problem is. You can do the talking whilst doing EFT™ for quicker and extra clearings. Make sure they are heard and understood and don't be patronising or dismissive.

When this belief was cleared, after the parts gave their cooperation, I could feel energy running all over my body which was very exciting and something I had never experienced before.

These parts can be:
- Intro vitro (in the womb)
- Inner child
- Childhood
- Adolescent
- Adult (split this into decades when investigating the age of the part)

EFT™ not working

If this doesn't appear to be working there would be various reasons for this:
- There are many aspects to the problem (discussed further on in this chapter)
- You haven't got the correct set up statement
- You may have a psychological reversal
- You are not clearing the patterns fully

So you need to go back to basics and write down your statements and then redo the routines making sure you over tap by a few days, speak out loudly (swear if appropriate!) and really feel what is going on. More about psychological reversals later in this chapter.

More advanced tapping routines

When you are more experienced you most probably will not need to use the Full Tapping Sequence as there are a variety of quick short forms. However, if the intensity number does not reduce, always return to the full tapping routine.

1. You can use the inner wrist point instead of tapping on all the finger points

2. You can exclude the setup statement and say different statements at each point. This is very effective and quick and I use this all the time:
   a. EB   I don't know why I can't lose weight
   b. SE   My metabolism is slow
   c. UE   I eat healthily
   d. UN   I exercise enough
   e. CH   Something is holding onto the weight
   f. CB   I must have water retention
   g. UA   I eat good protein
   h. TOP   I can't lose weight
3. Just think of the problem and keep tapping the KC point until you feel something release – this is the self sabotage point and I am told that people on the underground (subway in the States) are seen doing this all the time! Remember we sabotage our weight loss all the time!

Psychological Reversal

As I have mentioned before, the biggest turning point in my life was when I asked myself if I wanted to lose weight and the answer came back as a resounding NO! This, I was later to discover, is called a PSYCHOLOGICAL REVERSAL and it doesn't matter how hard you tap or work on yourself, the problem will always return.

What is PR?
PR, or Psychological Reversal to give it its full title, is when the work that is being undertaken does not stay changed. It's as though any changes are rejected because they are perceived as not being useful. It reverts back to what it was previously.

This can often be seen in clients who say:
- "Every time I start something I NEVER EVER finish it. I've always been like that!" or
- "I am always on a diet and lose the weight then put it all back on again."

Is there a test for PR?
Yes, you can test for PR using your diagnostic tools, muscle testing, dowsing and intuition. Whilst muscle testing or dowsing or using intuition you simply ask the question of the subconscious mind:

- "Does Rebecca's subconscious mind want to lose the weight?"
- "Does Rebecca's subconscious mind want her to change?"
- "Does Rebecca's subconscious mind want to stay in this relationship?"

Simple straightforward 'YES' or 'NO' response questions are asked of the subconscious mind.

What happens?

What happens is that the subconscious mind, which is stronger than the conscious mind, gives the correct answer by means of muscle testing or dowsing or intuition.

Can it be corrected?

YES

During the Set Up when you tap on the KC point, you are actioning the changes in the subconscious mind which are holding the PR in reverse/stuck mode. This works in 85% of cases automatically, simply by tapping the KC point during Set Up, PLUS you have the correct phrase.

Alternatively use the KC point and whilst thinking of the problem just keep tapping until you feel some kind of release – this doesn't have to be part of an EFT™ session.

In the other 15% when change or release does not take place, this shows that more advanced techniques are required. To release it you need to decide which one of the following statements is causing your PR and then tap continually on the KC point until you can feel it release. You will most probably have to do many rounds of EFT™ as well. This may take some days to do but is well worth the effort.

Reasons for PR can be for:
- It is not safe for me to lose weight
- It is not safe for others if I lose weight
- If I lose weight I will lose my identity
- Last time I lost weight I was abused /got pregnant / my husband left me/ I got too much attention from men
- I don't deserve to lose weight

- I am not worthy of losing weight
- If I lose weight I will have to get a job, move, have sex etc
- I am frightened of change/being slim/of everything

Simple physical tapping points

If you have a particular physical problem you can simply tap a point without the set up statement – you can do it anywhere and at anytime. Your subconscious knows what you are thinking about and associates the tapping with the problem:

Appetite overeating	UA
Allergies	Gamut
Anorexia Nervosa	UE
Appetite cycles	UE
Appetite lack off	UA
Appetite disorders	UE
Constipation	IF
Digestion of fats	SE
Diabetes	UA
Digestion of food	UA, IF
Endocrine imbalances	CB
Fluid retention	Gamut
Hormonal imbalance	CB
Hypoglycemia	UA
Lymphatic problems	Gamut
Menopause	CH
Nutrient absorption	KC
Night sweats	LF
Overeating	UA
Weight problems	UE, UA

The constipation short routine is brilliant and I use it every day.

Excellent for increasing the METABOLISM – whoopee!

This is an EFT™ routine that is purely designed to improve the working of the metabolism, but it can be used for any organ or metabolic process that is not working properly. You should use it every day to keep your metabolism working in peak condition. This can also be used on any other part of the body that is not functioning at 100%.

The Routine

1. What level in percentage is your metabolism functioning now? Let a number come to you or simply guess (which is one way of allowing your unconscious mind telling you what it actually is).
2. First round of tapping: "Even though my body only runs at xx percent, I deeply love and accept my body"
1. This clears out the most obvious blockages to the whole process and this takes you to the next step
2. Second round of tapping: "I want to release everything that slows my metabolism down and I deeply love and accept myself" (you can use body if you feel it is more appropriate)
3. Third round of tapping: "I want to repair everything that slows my metabolism/body down and I deeply love and accept myself"
4. Fourth round of tapping: "My metabolism is now working at 100% and is burning off my calories and I am getting slimmer every day and I LOVE MY METABOLISM". If your metabolism is only working at 60% please do not go straight to 100%. I would suggest increasing by 10% until you get to 100%

Looking into the future and tapping in the positive

You can use EFT™ for what you want to happen in the future and this works on reprogramming your belief system. However, this time the SUDS are normally given from 0 being no belief to 10 being total belief in yourself and are called SUBS (B being for Belief) So the reading goes up rather than down. These are the sorts of phrases you can use and you might find that the numbers take a while to creep up so I would use them several times every day, sometimes even for life. You don't need to put the affirmation at the end because the step up statement is normally an affirmation.

For example:

- I weigh (insert what you want to weigh) and that's what I weigh*
- My set point is ……….
- I am confident, healthy and sexy
- That new job is mine

*I would certainly use this set up several times a day, every day. You are programming your subconscious with what you want to weigh

Identifying links to traumas to find out what set you thinking you had a weight problem

It is a good idea to sit down with a chart of all traumas and life problems. From there work out what these traumas have installed in your subconscious that may be causing you problems today and tap on those problems, relating back to the trauma. Very often you find lots of other problems collapsing when you get back to the original root of the problem.

Even if your weight is linked to past lives or another problem, it may have been something that happened in this life that suddenly made your weight a problem (in my case it was becoming attuned to Reiki healing). These could be:

- Sexual abuse/rape
- Always being called chubby or chunky
- Sibling rivalry
- Having a mother that never loved you
- Miscarriage
- Divorce
- Death of a loved one
- Redundancy

From your chart work out which was the first incident that caused you a problem for your weight. Compile the setup phrase to include both incident and your weight problem. Listen to your insights and intuition as the set up phrase may need rewording several times to combine all the aspects of a problem. Then tap on the other incidents until they are all clear. You will then find that your relationship with your weight will change dramatically.

Different aspects

This is easier to explain with a snake phobia which I have had. I could tap on a phobia of snakes and it would reduce my SUDS level but I doubt whether it would go to zero because there are a lot of **aspects** to the problem. For example I don't like:

- The way their head moves
- The way their tongue moves and seems to twitch
- The way they slither over the floor
- The small matter of being poisonous!

- Their skin and texture
- The fact that some of them are enormous!
- Their beady eyes

I could tap on the first one and this may not be my major fear, so once again the SUDS level will not reduce quickly. So you need to put a SUDS number by each one to ensure that you tap on and collapse the most important one – and you may even find that the others don't need much tapping!

The way their head moves	10
The way their tongue moves and seems to twitch	10
The way they slither over the floor	8
The small matter of being poisonous!	7
Their skin and texture	5
The fact that some of them are enormous!	3
Their beady eyes	8

So from my SUDS level I would then have to work out which one that scored 10 was more important than the other – the best way is to do SUDS from zero to 100 or if they both come out at 100 then use your intuition. Tap on and clear to 0 the one with the most emotion and then work through the list in order. It is then quite a good idea to tap on 'everything else about a snake that I haven't covered' to catch all those other aspects that you haven't covered. However, the subconscious is very clever and it knows that snakes can be dangerous so it will remind you to have caution and not to put your hands in a pit of poisonous snakes!

So weight problems could have these aspects:

I will lose my identity if I lose weight	10
I will get too much attention and be harassed if I am slim	9
It is too hard to lose weight and I will fail	8
It is easier not to try than to fail	5
I may have to go out and find a new job	5
Everything else about my weight I have missed	4

Please remember that one problem normally has many aspects.

Testing

After you have tapped on a subject and got it to 0 it is a good idea to check the outcome now and in the future, as sometimes aspects may return if you think or concentrate on them. So after doing the snake phobia go to a zoo or handle a snake and see what comes up. Do you have any fear or have other aspects now been shown to you for you to tap on?

Other examples of testing for weight:
- Hold a bag of crisps or a bar of chocolate and see how you feel – do you want to eat it or are you quite happy to leave it alone?
- If you have tapped on reducing your appetite put a big plate of food in front of you – do you want to eat it all or do you want to leave some?

Instant emotional release

If you are having an emotional crisis there are some points you can press which will help release the problem – the secret is holding two points together and either press gently or tap, whichever your intuition leads to.
- Press collar bone and under arm together
- Press thumb on the gamut point and the index finger on the karate spot

The second option can be used if the first option is hard for you to do.

Cravings

Usually when you have a craving it is because either you are deficient in vitamins or your body is telling you that you need that food. There was an article recently that showed that a woman craved lettuce and was eating up to eight a day. Her husband was a doctor and when he investigated it he discovered that she had a particular type of cancer and the minerals and vitamins in this type of lettuce were shown to shrink the tumour. Or it could be that you are trying to give yourself love, praise, attention or to stuff down emotions – or that you have no sweetness in your life and you are trying to fill that gap.

I also have a section in this book showing that if you crave crisps you may have an adrenal problem so you really need to listen to your body and what it is trying to tell you.

To reduce cravings always take the mineral chromium. Then use EFT™ every time you have a craving until it is eliminated.

Addictions

If you have an addictive personality you most probably have addictions to certain types of food. You can also have them even if you don't have that type of personality because the food industries pay millions of pounds in research to make food look and taste absolutely fantastic. They fill it full of additives that make it addictive and even look at the crunch of an apple and a crisp to make it more desirable.

That is why our food is so full of added things that shouldn't be there. I bought a fish pie and when I looked at the ingredients it contained pork fat. When I rang the company and asked why (as I don't eat meat) they informed me that it made it taste better. It certainly didn't taste better to me!

Don't feel that you are weak – the fat industry is trying to grab you to buy their products.

Using a technique like EFT™ can eliminate addictions quite easily and simply and you can use it at any time, especially if you are tempted!

Habits

It is supposed to take twenty eight days to form a habit but believe me it is much quicker than that. You know yourself that if you have a coffee and add a biscuit this becomes a habit in a couple of days and you almost shake when you try and stop it. However, it can take twenty eight days to stop a habit and you do need to be extremely strong with yourself. Using a technique like EFT™ is far the best way to deal with this and use it constantly until the habit of wanting and eating the food has gone. Also you any time an emotional problem comes up, you feel bored or you saddening have a desire to overeat and your resolve has gone! Also use it daily on your willpower which needs constant help

Why these issues can have their roots in an emotional issue

When I have been working with clients very often there is another reason why a person is additive to or craves food or alcohol. When you clear the first layer there is usually an issue that is causing the problem so this is why you need to keep going with EFT™ until you can sit with a plate full of what you crave or are addictive to for hours without wanting to eat the lot!!

Very often overeating is associated with the following:
- Being born by C section
- Being put in an incubator
- Not being nurtured by your mother
- Being given food to shut you up or as a treat
- Grief and loss
- No sweetness in your life
- Lack of money
- Abandonment/Rejection
- Stuffing down an emotional issue
- Not feeling safe
- Subconscious issue of not going to survive unless you overeat (caveman!)
- Fear of getting close to people
- Disgust with yourself for overeating or being fat
- Comfort food for problems such as bullying or unhappiness
- Not getting attention or love from anybody so you get this from food
- Boredom
- To cope with emotions
- Obsession with food
- Peer pressure
- Additive personality
- Low self esteem and confidence, lack of self belief and self worth
- Family problems of overeating or gluttony

Working with yourself or with a client

In my experience weight problems have very little do with food and have much deeper origins. Not including subjects like karma and past lives, there is a reason why the client is putting on weight, holding onto it or regaining back all the lost weight. So it is very important to get to the core issues of the problem (and there are normally more than one). Joanne (my client) worked on all her issues and lost weight quite easily and has since maintained her weight as she has no reason to put it back on again!

Very often these are to do with the following:
- Issues with self-worth/not being deserving
- Starving for attention/stuffing down words or feelings
- Not feeling lovable
- Self punishment and suffering patterns
- Not being in control of their life/boredom
- Fear of being slim for various reasons
- Protection against attention
- Because of what happened the last time they were slim

In addition, it is essential that a full case history is taken – a bit like being a detective really! When I worked with called Joanne, this is was what uncovered:

1. She felt she wasn't worthy of reaching her goals – she didn't deserve to reach her target weight
2. She needed the extra weight as protection against men who would 'harass' her for being slim and beautiful
3. She didn't feel lovable enough (please note that this comes up a lot)

She had never felt worthy or lovable. Her parents wanted a son and were disappointed when they had had a girl. She could feel their disappointment and this was reflected in their behaviour which was cold and unloving. Therefore she was starving for attention.

Joanne found that the weight started to drop off as her self-worth rose and her fear of men fell. She could feel when she was full and other subliminal messages came to her automatically such as 'clean your plate because of the starving children in the world'. We have all heard that one, methinks!

She also used EFT™ to stop sabotaging herself. As I mentioned earlier, Joanne felt she never got enough recognition or praise when she did something right, so she was 'starving' for attention. Self-esteem issues can be the core of self- sabotage and every aspect needs to be worked on. Statements must include self-esteem issues and deprivation issues around love and attention for the weight loss to be permanent. In my case my mother controlled me all my life and it was essential that the power came back to me and I gave myself permission to do it my way.

- Even though I feel discouraged by how much weight I need to lose, I choose to reward myself every step of the way
- Even though I feel deprived that I can't eat what I want like other people, I choose to reward myself in other ways
- Even though I feel threatened by the attention of men, I choose to feel secure
- Even though I'm afraid to be successful because I'll be too different, I claim success now
- Even though they have tried to control me all my life, I choose to take back my power
- Even though I feel deeply resentful, I choose to accept my feelings
- Even though I'm using my weight challenge as a way to get in my own way, I deeply and completely love and accept all of me
- Even though there was never enough love for me, I choose to feel safe now
- Even though I am not loveable enough, I love and accept myself

Chapter 22:
LIFE COACHING AND OTHER THERAPIES

YESTERDAY, TOMORROW AND TODAY

There are two days in every week about which we should not worry.
Two days that should be kept free from fear and apprehension.

One of these days is yesterday with its mistakes and cares,
its faults and blunders, its aches and pains.
Yesterday has passed forever beyond our control.
All the money in the world cannot bring back yesterday.
We cannot undo a single act we performed.
We cannot erase a single word we said. Yesterday is gone.

The other day we should not worry about is tomorrow.
With its possible adversities, its burdens, its large promise and
poor performance, tomorrow is also beyond our immediate control.
Tomorrow's sun will rise, either in splendour or behind a
mask of clouds, but it will rise.
Until it does, we have no stake in tomorrow, for it is yet unborn.

This leaves only one day - today.
Any person can fight the battle for just one day.
It is only when you and I add the burdens of those two awful eternities,
yesterday and tomorrow, that we break down.
It is not the experience of today that drives people mad.
It is the remorse of bitterness for something which happened yesterday
and the dread of what tomorrow may bring.

Let us therefore live but one day at a time.

Author Unknown

What is Life Coaching?

Life Coaching is mainly about setting realistic goals that you then adhere to. The reason I like life coaching is that it is positive, energetic and supportive and allows you to discover **and** manifest inner strengths (that you most probably didn't know that you had). Unlike most therapies, it looks to the future rather than the past and therefore it is a highly effective way of making tangible changes and moving forward in a relatively short period of time.

However, as you can see by my story, setting goals isn't the total answer. I am proof that you can set as many goals as you like, read them and act on them but if your self-sabotage is in full swing nothing will move forward until that self-sabotage is healed and released. So I would suggest that life coaching is carried out with EFT™ so you can release the issues as you go along, such as procrastination, not thinking you are good enough or any other reason that is stopping you.

But, by setting goals, I was able to keep a close check on my progress and knew when the time was right to try something new or investigate another avenue. Reading my goal plan enabled me to keep focused and motivated. The plan also helped me look at what I have achieved and congratulate myself on my progress, something that we often forget to do.

Being your own life coach

Start creating your own life coaching plan, identifying and writing down your goals. Use an excel spreadsheet or equivalent so you can easily monitor your progress. If it is all written down in a notebook, it might not be so easy to review.

Set specific goals
Normally your ideas of goals are in your head and a bit vague – you know roughly what you want to do but never seem to quite put it into practice. So be very specific and add the date by when you want this goal achieved:
1. How much weight do I want to lose?
2. When do I want to lose it by?
3. What dress size do I want to end up?
4. What particular areas do I want to tone up?
5. What cravings or addictions do I want to eliminate?
6. What eating plan do I want to follow for life?
7. What exercise plan do I want to follow for life?

Set measurable goals
You must be able to measure your goals otherwise you will never know whether you have reached them or not. So when reviewing them you will know if you have to amend them in anyway.

1. Once a month check weight, body fat, clothes size and generally how you feel
2. How is your eating plan going?
3. How is your exercise plan going?
4. How are your alternative therapies working – do you need to try something else?

Set realistic goals

You are not going to lose 10lbs in a weekend, whatever the advert says, especially if you have a problem with your metabolism. Remember that you have to get your body working and performing correctly before weight loss will occur.

There are no unrealistic goals only unrealistic deadlines!

1. How long is it going to take to get your endocrine system to work?
2. How long is it going to take to get used to your eating plan/exercise routine?

Set short term and long term goals

You must make a list of both short term and long term goals. Your long term goal may be to lose weight and keep it off. But this will be made up of masses of short term goals.

Set the following goals:

1. Your ultimate long term goal/s (there can be more than one)
2. Yearly goals
3. Three monthly goals
4. Monthly goals
5. Weekly goals
6. Daily goals

To have this mix of goals means that you know that you are on track. If you slip, you can identify it immediately and make the necessary adjustments. That is why you must read your goals daily. Not only does this make them real and attainable, but you can see at a glance if your goals are not going to plan. This keeps your motivation level very high and motivation is the key!

Set big goals where appropriate

Make goals scary and exciting and don't think you can't strive for what you really dream of, not just what you want to achieve. So think big, dream and fantasise about these goals. Have you always wanted to travel the world or become an author? The only person stopping you doing this is you so make these your big goals.

1. What job would you really like to do?
2. How much money would you really like to earn?
3. Who would you like to emulate?
4. How healthy do you want to be?
5. How slim would you like to be?

Establish the emotional reasons why you don't want to achieve your goals

By reading your goals daily you can quickly identify the emotional reasons why you don't want to achieve your goals. You will now be very familiar with EFT and Tapping and you can now immediately work on these issues, clear and resolve them. This is another important reason for keeping a journal to record all the positives, negative emotions and how you have dealt with them and moved on. Is it fear? Are you procrastinating? Do you think you are not good enough? All these reasons will stop your goals becoming reality.

Write down your list of goals in a positive manner
Now you need to start writing down your goals. They must be positive, using "I" and in the present tense:

1. I am slim and attractive
2. I am eating healthily
3. I am exercising effectively
4. I am taking my supplements daily

If you feel these aren't true use something like:

1. I am getting slimmer every day
2. I am getting more and more toned every day
3. I am eating more healthily every day
4. I remember to take my supplements every day

Read those goals
The main reason that most peoples' goals fail is that they don't read them enough. They set them up and then tuck them in a folder waiting for them to miraculously work! You need to keep your goals with you and read them at least once a day, more if you can. Think about them, visualise them, feel them and make them real.

Read the goals as if they have been achieved. If any doubts creep in, immediately use EFT™ to resolve and heal them.

Counselling

The reasons people come to counselling are as varied as the people themselves. Often, clients have encountered distressing or stressful experiences, or situations which they'd like to talk about in a safe setting. These might include bereavement, separation or other major life transitions, or experiences from the past such as in childhood. Others seek help in dealing with specific psychological or behavioural traits which they'd like to alter, for instance compulsive thoughts or difficulties relating to people.

Some people seek counselling to help them explore a general feeling that their lives are not quite right or to cope with feelings of depression, anxiety or self- esteem problems. Others look to counselling as part of their effort to discover or create meaning in their lives.

Very often people think they are alone and nobody has ever experienced what they are going through. However, it is good to have somebody listen who is totally non-judgmental - especially about health and weight problems, where people judge us all the time. Health and weight is also a subject where people assume that they are experts and come up with various (unhelpful) suggestions like "I know why you are fat because you eat too much / you eat too little / you don't eat breakfast".

Counselling has been available for decades now and has been used very successfully, although resolving problems can take years. This is why I would recommend that counselling is used with other therapies such as EFT™, as the emotional problems are resolved, healed and released far quicker. Make a few calls to counsellors and use your intuition to choose the one you can relate to – or you can book an appointment with me!

By using something like EFT™ to release the stuck emotions, you can become your own counsellor. EFT™ is now being used by counsellors and psychotherapists to get better and quicker results from their sessions, so why not harness the power of this yourself?

Being your own counsellor

Sit down with a pen and a piece of paper. Say out loud to yourself "I can't lose weight because" and then talk until you can't think of anything else to say and write down what comes up. This could be something like:

- I have too much weight to lose, the task is too big. I will not achieve it and give up after a week
- My resolve is not good and I will fail
- I am frightened of failure
- I feel safe when I am fat
- If I lose weight I might lose my identity

Then use EFT™ until all these feelings have been released. It may take several days. When you feel 'clearer' repeat the exercise over a month until you start losing weight. This is a good technique if you reach a plateau because, remember, you are creating that with a block so you need to release the block before can resume your weight loss.

My experience

I trained to be a counsellor and I have to say that I was slightly wary of the whole process, especially having trained in life coaching, EFT™ and various other meridian therapies. Although I think it is good to talk things through, problems and issues need to be resolved and you need to move forward, otherwise what is the point?

If not done correctly, counselling can make people more aware of their problems, or very self-centred – that is why I go for the quicker release type of techniques, such as EFT™.

I nearly got attacked by the students when I said that I thought stress was the most commonly overused word in the English dictionary. People now talk about going to the supermarket and dropping the kids off to school as stressful. Ten years ago we would have said that it was a hassle or unpleasant – goodness knows what these people are going to do if something really stressful happens in their life, like a loved one dying or bankruptcy.

The other worrying thing was when the symptoms of stress were written on the board, everybody in the class (excluding me!) said that they had them – all of them. There are masses of techniques available for stress which people don't seem to be using. Perhaps it's because they like to wallow in their stress or they have become addicted to stress. This all made me very wary of using a counsellor, as these were the counsellors of the future!

During a role playing session, one young student, who had lost several elderly relatives and was attending private counselling herself, was asked by somebody on the course why she was upset. She replied that that although they were elderly, they were very close to her, it was her first experience of death and she was finding it difficult to come to terms with it. The other student said "Well they were old, so why are you bothered?" I hope I never get her as a counsellor!

Hypnosis and hypnotherapy

The brain operates in four general states which include full conscious awareness (Beta), the hypnotic state (Alpha), the dream state (Theta), and the sleeps state (Delta). Full conscious awareness is where which we spend most of our waking hours. In this state, our mind is attentive and uses logic to reason, evaluate and make decisions. Unfortunately, when making life changes, the conscious mind often gets in the way.

In the hypnotic state, the doorway between the conscious and the subconscious is opened, memories become easily accessible and new positive and life changing information is stored. In the hypnotic state, you are not really 'thinking' but more 'experiencing' without questioning, without critical judgment or analysis, like when you watch a film, and the hypnotherapist can then make positive suggestions that are very likely to 'stick' - precisely because your conscious mind is not getting in the way.

In hypnotherapy, a deep state of relaxation is achieved through concentrating on what the hypnotherapist is saying. When you are in a trance-like state, the use of imagery and positive suggestions can help you to imagine and actually experience yourself in the future, as you desire to be. This makes the changes you want in your life to happen much faster and with less resistance.

Hypnotherapy is particularly effective for addictive habits such as overeating, weight and emotional problems, as well as for stress control.

My experiences

I use hypnotherapy in many ways on clients:
* For past life regression

- Installing positive messages into the subconscious mind for self-esteem and weight loss
- Persuading the body to eat slowly
- Encouraging the body to want exercise
- Picturing yourself thin and how you would like to look
- Reminding the subconscious to think twice before eating food or having that glass of wine (people don't seem to count wine as calories)
- Encouraging self-love and good body image
- Reinforcing your positive points
- Setting up negative feelings for foods etc that you want to cut out, such as chocolate or crisps
- Eliminating intolerances, addictions, habits and cravings

I will also EFT™ when a client is IN a relaxed state to reinforce the positive messages that are being given to the subconscious.

Self-hypnosis

One of the ways that hypnotherapy really interests me is in the form of self-hypnosis – you can put yourself under very quickly and simply to either sort out a problem, reinforce positive messages and to handle pain – this technique is excellent for handling pain.

This simple self-hypnosis routine brings together several different psychological principles. You might feel a little bit drowsy immediately after doing this exercise but don't worry, this is normal and will go away after a few minutes as you become grounded. However, you should avoid driving until you get your orientation back.

Meditation text

This simple meditation will help you become familiar with relaxing, breathing and repeating affirmations.

Find a place to relax where you are unlikely to be disturbed. Assume a position in which you can comfortably relax, either lying down or seated. Choose a 'trigger word' which will help you to relax, such as 'relax'; you will repeat this at the beginning of each deep breath. Choose an affirmation or positive suggestion which you can repeat to yourself, such as' I love myself or' I am happy', 'I am a size 14' or 'I have released all my weight', or anything else that you want to programme your subconscious with. Finally, visualise a relaxing scene, perhaps lying on the beach or sitting in the garden. If you have problems visualising a scene simply imagine that you are being enveloped by a soothing, shapeless cloud of coloured mist.

Imagine that your body is divided into three sections which you will relax in turn: firstly, from your waist down to your feet, secondly, your torso and arms and thirdly, your head and neck.

- Allow your eyelids to fall shut, take a few moments just to unwind, focus on your breathing, clear your mind and get comfortable.
- Take a deep breath in. Hold your breath for about ten or fifteen seconds before letting out a deep sigh and relaxing your whole body. Say your trigger word as you exhale. Allow your breathing to return to normal for a few moments and just be aware of how relaxed your body now feels.
- Breathe in again, in the same way, and this time relax your lower body, from your waist down to your feet, as you exhale and repeat the trigger word.
- Take another deep breath, relaxing your chest, back and arms as you exhale.
- Breathe in again and relax your head, neck and face as you breathe out.
- Finally, to catch any tension that might have returned to your body, relax your whole body again as you breath out. If you want you can also use this breath to imagine that you are expelling any emotional or mental tension.
- Take a few moments to settle and allow your breathing to return to normal and your mind to become empty, tranquil and quiet.
- If necessary, allow your attention to be drawn to any part of your body where tension has returned. Imagine that it is a puff of coloured smoke and visualise it being blown away by a warm breeze.
- Now visualise yourself standing at the top of a flight of ten stairs or steps, at the bottom of which is your relaxing place. Slowly descend the steps one at a time, counting from ten all the way down to zero as you do so. Try to feel yourself sinking down deeper toward a light trance with each step you take.
- When you arrive at the bottom of the steps visualise yourself entering into your relaxing scene. Take a few minutes to try to get a feel for the scene, take a note of the colours and shapes

which you can see, and any sounds. Allow yourself to let go completely and enjoy the pleasant feelings of physical relaxation and mental calm.

- Now, repeat your affirmation to yourself in your own time, for as long as you want. Remember to be aware of your imaginary tone of voice.

- When you are finished, take time to settle again and to enjoy the feelings of calmness and confidence which your affirmation has given you.

- When you are ready, count from one up to five. Open your eyes, clench your fists and give your arms and legs a shake to wake yourself up again.

Your own script

Another way of self-hypnosis is to go into a trance and make up your own script.

1. Determine what you want to achieve before going into a trance It could be affirmations such as 'I accept that my legs/bum/breasts aren't perfect, but I still like and respect myself', 'I want to stop craving crisps', or 'my wrinkles are disappearing and my skin is smoother'.

2. Tell yourself you are going to do self-hypnosis. Make yourself comfortable and close your eyes. Begin slowly and, mentally count down from ten to one, saying each descending number as you breathe out slowly. For maximum relaxation, try to make each out-breath last at least three times longer than your in-breath. If you are not totally relaxed on reaching the count of one, simply repeat the process.

3. Next, repeat your mantra, either out loud or under your breath, for as long as it takes for your mood to change. Imagine yourself slim, turn and notice how flat your stomach is, how toned your bottom is. Smooth your hands over your hips and see how you smile with satisfaction. If there is any negativity or resistance, gather it up and let it release out of your body – nothing is going to stop you. This is you.

4. You can always wake from the trance as quickly as you want but the best method is to slowly and mentally count up from one to ten and then open your eyes. For best results practice every day – remember - practice, practice, practice and then it becomes second nature.

Going into hypnosis quickly

When you are familiar with the hypnosis techniques you can go into hypnosis very quickly. Programme going into hypnosis with either a trigger word or physical movement. So when you want to go into hypnosis quickly just set the intent and state your trigger word or movement. You can do this when you are in a queue in a supermarket, whilst stationary in a traffic jam or anywhere else that you have some time. When you are ready to come out of hypnosis use the same trigger word or movement.

Pain control

When you have reached the point where you are relaxed say, as you snap your fingers, "In future when I snap my fingers all the pain I am feeling will be gone". This is setting up the trigger in your subconscious for the future. So when you get a headache, snap your fingers and see what happens!

Self-help CDs

I have mentioned in other chapters that there are masses of CDs you can purchase to help yourself lose weight and feel better and these are listed in Appendix A. The ones I recommend are from Paul McKenna.

Don't forget a subliminal computer programme to help you on your way as well. I have one on my computer at all times. There is a variety on the internet and I downloaded one that was free and it is excellent.

Neuro-linguistic programming (NLP)

NLP is a fantastic method for changing behaviour and provides you with the tools and skills for your future development. NLP is about self-discovery and exploring how and why you tick and, if necessary, how to change your belief system.

NLP describes the fundamental dynamics between mind (neuro) and language (linguistic) and how their interplay affects our body and behaviour (programming). When you first start to use NLP, the terminology can be very complicated and confusing. So I have listed below the easiest, but most successful I feel, NLP techniques

Anchoring:

This is where you use a technique to anchor a time when you felt good about yourself and to reinforce this feeling in the future. So think about a time in the past where you felt slim, happy or excited and make this feeling really big, colourful and deep. Then use a trigger that can anchor that feeling in your subconscious for instant recall in the future – it could be a snap of the fingers, a pinch or turning on a light switch. Keep repeating this until you really feel the feeling and it is so easy to go back into that feeling. So in the future when you need a boost, use your trigger (snap your fingers for example) and instantly that happy memory will be recalled and you will be transported back to that time and then bring that happy feeling into now and the future.

Mirroring:

You may have heard of this technique before. It is used as an interview or sales technique, where you mirror the voice and the actions of the person that is opposite you. If, say, you are generally loud and chatty it could put the interviewer or customer off, so if they are quietly spoken you become quietly spoken. This works on the theory that people respond to somebody better if they are like themselves.

Moving things around:

If something is bothering you, a person for example, imagine them in a frame right in front of your eyes and make it big and colourful. Then make the picture very small, grey and change the person to a comedy figure such as Daffy Duck! Then start moving the picture around from your front to your back and finish with the picture at the back – this confuses the subconscious and it loses where it has stored the original picture. Then see the picture disappear completely. Now think about that person and you will find that your feelings have become neutral. If they haven't, repeat the exercise.

Visualisation

The technical explanation is that visualisation takes place when the mind reproduces an image, even though no source for the image is present for the eyes to see. In my opinion visualisation is a wonderful technique to use in your everyday life.

During my self-sabotage era I could recover my kidneys from not working to working within five minutes by visualising everything that was hurting my kidneys being removed and then being soothed by green light. I then visualised my kidneys working correctly with the water passing through them and feeding my bladder.

Another of my visualisations is how I always wanted to look – that is slim, attractive, in a red suit, with long blonde curly hair. I visualise this image all the time and can easily step into it and make the visualisation real. Slowly the figure becomes full size and is standing right in front of me. Much to my amusement, the Ann in the red suit started to step into me a bit at a time every time I released more stuff until only a small part of my bottom stuck out – it was hilarious!

Visualise how you want to look and repeat it so often that you can recall this picture at any time. Imagine the picture to be full size and look at the new you and make it so real. Then step into the new you and become one and see how it feels.

Visualise yourself eating small portions and exercising - and enjoying both.

Visualise your organs working by releasing anything that is dark and replacing it with colour and movement.

The more you do this the more alive this picture will become and the more you will believe that it is how you are going to be. During my years of self-sabotage, this is the one thing that kept me going. I KNEW I was going to become that girl, in that vibrant red suit.

Rewrite your past
When you link into your past and you connect with events that made you unhappy, you revert back to victim mode which will reduce your vibration. Most people did not have an idyllic childhood so you are not alone. However, what you can do is rewrite the past – I did this and within 7 days I couldn't think about events that had upset me before and the feeling of having a loving and supportive childhood started to change me and my self esteem rose. So try to do this daily until you feel a change and then do it a couple of times a week – or if you feel you are slipping back into old painful feelings. You need to go back before you were conceived so I have prepared a small script but you must use your own words and what you would have liked to have happened.

"My parents were very much in love and wanted a baby so when I was conceived I was wanted and loved. The pregnancy was so easy for my mother and myself and I could feel her love and support as I was growing. The birth was a wonderful experience and I was welcomed into the world by a great team and to the smiling faces of my mother

and father. As a child I was encouraged, supported, praised, loved and wanted. I was intelligent and quick to pick things up and I excelled at school. My parents asked my opinions and I felt that I was being taken seriously, I was being listened to and that my needs were met. Even when I didn't do so well in school I was praised and encouraged and I always felt worthy and good enough. I past my exams with ease and went on to have a fantastic well paid career. I was healthy with a fast metabolism and I was slim and attractive. I have an amazingly happy marriage and I am so happy and manifesting the life of my dreams".

Speak to your disease or stress

When you are ill very often your body is trying to tell you something and you need to listen to what it is saying otherwise you will get worse. The best way is to speak to your disease/stress so you can understand the main cause which means you can start to put it right. Perhaps you are stressed because your body is exhausted and you are being told to rest or change your job. There are many reasons and you may be surprised by the answer! Underactive thyroid problems are usually to do with not feeling safe with male attention or not being able to speak up for yourself. You need to sit quietly where you won't be disturbed and go into a meditative state. Perhaps light a candle and some incense to get you into the mood.

"Ask for your disease/stress to appear before you in front of you so you can see it. Thank it for coming and say that you want to understand why you are ill and that you are also willing to start healing what the main problem is. Listen to what it has to say and don't argue or start disagreeing with it remember it is trying to help you. Ask it what the original cause was and what can you do now to heal it and feel better. You may be told you are allergic to something, or that something is poisoning you, or that some deep emotional trauma needs to be healed before you can heal, that the illness is keeping you safe (this is the case with ME as ME is fear of living) or you may be working too hard without proper nourishment and you may have to cut your hours or take supplements. Thank the disease/stress for its help and information and promise that you will connect with it weekly to ensure that you are doing enough to help heal".

Speak to your parallel or future self

We are always being told to visualise ourselves as if what we wanted had happened and I do agree with this. However, I did this for 17 years on my new slim figure and it didn't make a difference because I had patterns and karma that was stopping it happening. This exercise really takes it to the next level where you meet your future/parallel self and merge with them. You need to sit quietly where you won't be disturbed and go into a meditative state. Perhaps light a candle and some incense to get you into the mood.

"You are feeling very relaxed and you are walking along a corridor where there are multiple doors. Behind one of these doors is your parallel or future self who has released all the negative beliefs, karma, past lives and everything else that is stopping you moving forward and you are dying to meet them! You instinctively know which door to go through so push the door open. On the other side you see yourself exactly as you want to look, doing exactly what you want to do. You run over to them and you embrace. Instantly they start removing blocks and anything they can see that is blocking you. They are whispering new positive beliefs into your ears and your whole body is feeling alive with positive vibrations. You then merge with your parallel/future self and feel how good it is to have the body and the life of your dreams. Spend a few minutes feeling like this and then come back to reality knowing that this is happening now. Redo this exercise as often as you can to reinforce the healing".

Chapter 23:
OTHER THERAPIES AND TECHNIQUES FOR WEIGHT LOSS

In the time that I spent getting answers to my problems, I spent over fifteen years visiting therapists and spent in excess of £250,000. This puts me in a great position to advise you as to whether these therapies work for weight loss or not. Obviously, what works for one doesn't necessarily work for another but I wish somebody could have pointed me in the right direction when I first set out on my path.

We have already talked about the techniques and therapies that I recommend such as homeopathy, herbs, Emotional Freedom Technique and crystals. The following treatments are ones that I have selected out of thousands of different therapies that I have tried and from which I have gained considerable benefit. That is not to say that the other therapies are not affective, they are, but just not for weight loss.

The treatments that I think that everybody should try are marked with an asterisk, showing that I highly recommend them.

Reflexology

Reflexology is massaging points on the feet and the hands that relate to organs of the body and this can either be done by a therapist or by yourself if you are just using a couple of points. This is an ideal treatment for weight loss because you can stimulate the points for the hypothalamus, pituitary, pineal and thyroid glands, either on your feet or on your hands. This will increase the workings of these organs and hopefully stimulate the metabolism to help you lose weight. You can also activate the lymphatic system, kidneys and bladder and any other organ that is not performing to its maximum potential, such as the pancreas or gallbladder.

Either book a consultation with a reflexology practitioner who has been recommended to you or is in a successful practice – you really need to go to somebody who is experienced not somebody that has just qualified. Ask them to then show you all the relevant points on your hands and feet and how to stimulate them so you can continue to treat yourself at home, or you could buy yourself a good book (there are plenty on Amazon) and study the book yourself. To begin with though, it would be better to see a practitioner so that they can work on the whole body to get you into balance before you concentrate on the endocrine organs.

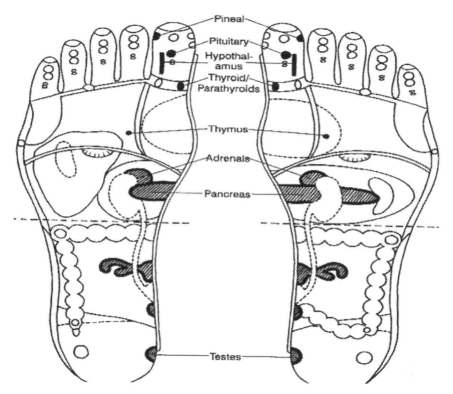

Acupuncture

I have to say that as far as I was concerned acupuncture had no effect on my weight but it did help with releasing the water and healing my kidney meridian lines. Acupuncture is a very old therapy that has been used in China for thousands of years and has now become popular, even being recommended by doctors. It has tremendous effects on lots of issues such as bone and muscles and on chronic fatigue. An acupuncturist will put very small, fine needles into specific points on the body's meridian lines.

However, some people have had some success with auricular (ear) acupuncture and have had a device fitted to the inside of their ear, similar to a staple. When you crave food you rub this device and the idea is that your appetite disappears. Because the device is semi-permanent for however long you have agreed with your therapist, it is supposed to dull the appetite all the time as well.

Acupressure

Acupressure is similar to acupuncture but instead of a needle you rub the specific point with your thumb or relevant fingers. As with reflexology, there are various specific points around the body which relate to organs and problems, so you can have specific points for kidneys or for water retention.

I would suggest that you buy a good book that gives you lots of examples of where these points are and how to access them. As you are doing this yourself it means that you can massage these points every day.

Cranial sacral therapy*

Cranial sacral therapy is an excellent treatment and I am lucky to have the most amazing practitioner who has sorted out my imbalances which helped me lose weight. Nobody had picked up that my parasympathetic and sympathetic system was on panic alert and was flooding my body with adrenaline and cortisol.

The official explanation is that cranial sacral therapy works on many different levels and influences many different structures within the body. It influences the musculo-skeletal system, the nervous system, the cardiovascular-vascular system, the immune system, the organs, the connective tissues, the fluids and the energy systems of the body. It therefore has widespread and profound effects on conditions affecting all of these systems.

I cannot recommend this treatment highly enough and it is excellent for children as well.

Hands on Healing

I am a great believer in hands on healing, and although I don't think that it is necessarily brilliant for weight loss, it is excellent for balancing the body and making you feel relaxed and absolutely wonderful. It can also bring issues to the surface that need healing.

Only you can heal yourself - hands on healing kicks in the body's own healing mechanism which in turn will start healing all the areas that need attention, for whatever reason. So always be very wary of people who say they can heal you – the only person who can heal you is you yourself.

Again, I would go to somebody that is recommended or has been established for a long time. Because of my problems with Reiki, I wouldn't want you to discount this form of healing. However, if you were to decide to go down the Reiki path and become attuned to being a healer, I would very thoroughly research the Reiki Masters who would be doing the training and make sure that you have a good rapport.

Manual lymphatic drainage

This is a type of massage that works solely on the lymphatic system of the body. MLD activates the lymph glands and pushes the lymph around the body. To begin with you normally have to have a treatment every couple of days to kick start your system but when you are finished, you have no puffiness and once swollen ankles are as slim as anything – I found it truly amazing – especially the puffiness around the eyes disappearing.

This treatment is also used heavily in cancer cases where a lymph node has been removed and with a condition called lymph oedema which causes swelling of the legs, ankles, stomach, hands and fingers. However, it is not used if you currently have cancer.

I have a MLD once a month now just to keep things ticking over. I would highly recommend this treatment if you have any form of oedema or water retention.

Hair Analysis*

When I was seeing a rather pompous endocrinologist in London without much success, as the medication didn't work and he wouldn't listen to what I said, my friend said that he should do more tests and they would show up more of the problem and why the medication didn't work. So when he didn't do any more tests we were both perplexed! Then when a lady with whom I was working in the States said she wanted me to have my hair analysed I began to think this might be the breakthrough. To begin with I declined, as I had had hair analysis done before, for allergies etc, but I was told that this was very different – and believe me it was.

This laboratory analyses the minerals and vitamins in your hair and they can then ascertain how your thyroid and adrenals are working, how you are metabolising proteins and carbohydrates and generally how your body is working – it was truly amazing and like the missing link.

Of course it said that my thyroid and adrenals were dangerously low and that I didn't metabolise anything properly but it did say that my immune system was good and that was a relief. It made me realise I wasn't going mad and I now recommend that everybody I see in my clinic has their hair analysed to find out what is going wrong. In my case I was being poisoned by copper and calcium. You then get masses of useful and interesting information on how you can detox what is poisoning you and how to ensure that it doesn't happen again.

For more information on this please contact me and I will send you a form.

Universal Clay body wrap

When I had a beauty salon I used this type of body wrap with great success. You are covered in clay and wrapped in bandages – yes you do end up looking like a mummy! You then gently exercise for an hour. The clay removes the excess water and toxins and you can lose inches. I have to say that the clay was was more effective than any others I tried. This is a real boost when you are losing weight and it is a good idea to have one when you go on holiday.

Obviously if you put on a bit of weight some of the inches will go back on but it is good for a lift.

Vision board

This is a board (or folder) where you cut out pictures of what you desire and this would include your new body, your new clothes you will wear when you are slim and will also include your dream house, job, soul mate or car. Look at this board several times a day and make all the pictures real. Place the board where you can see it for most of the day. This will work with your meditation and hypnosis to create the life you would like. Talk to your vision board so you are sending the message of what you want out to the universe and you are making it real. Talk like it has already happened and this will also make it real.

Writing and speaking emotions out

One of the best ways to release emotions from yourself is to write the down and keep going until the emotional feelings have left you. If you have a problem with somebody it is a good idea to write them a letter detailing everything you think, read it out loud then print it out and burn it – it is not a good idea to send the letter to the person if you want to remain friends! Why not write a letter to your "fat" self explaining how you feel and asking for its cooperation in losing weight – it really does work.

If you can't seem to achieve what you want start off my saying "I can't lose weight because" and keep going until you can't think of anything else. It is a good idea to do this daily as more emotion will come up over night.

Declutter your life

It is very important that you declutter your friends, house, car and desk as you are decluttering your body and mind. If friends no longer serve let them go from your life with love – don't try and hold onto them. Get rid of ornaments that you no longer want and throw out things that you haven't used in a year – chances are you are never going to use it again!

Make sure that your house and car (and office) are clean and tidy as this makes for a clean and tidy mind. If you do this you will find that you lose weight faster.

Feng shui

Although Feng shui (the Chinese philosophical system of harmonizing the human existence with the surrounding environment) is not explained in this book, it would be a good idea to buy a book to ensure that your house and life are working in your favour, especially to release lack.

Cutting cords

Very often we have cords to people, situations and places – and this could be on the of the reasons you can't lose weight. These cords stop us being free as most of them are negative and are holding us back. This is why you can't totally forget a former partner or you still long for an old job, as you are still linked. You shouldn't have any cords to anything and this includes family and loved ones. We should all be free to enjoy each other's company and want to be friends, rather than having to be because of the cords.

So sit quietly and see if you can see any cords to the person or the situation and where they are going. Are they going to the heart, head or to an office? If you can't see where these cords are, don't worry as they will be cut anyway. So ask Archangel Michael to cut all the cords between you and everybody or everything with his sword. He should cut the ones in front of you, behind you, under you and over your head. Sit quietly and relax until you feel this process is completed and then ask to be filled with healing energy. To start with you need to do this exercise every day for a week and then once weekly. This is when developing your intuition helps because you immediately know when you have a new cord that needs cutting. Somebody that you are connected to might not want you to lose weight so they are sabotaging your efforts – yes this really does happen!

A great friend of mine had horrendous family problems and felt like she was too attached to them. Of course she was via her cords. She completed this process and even after one session she felt so much better and lighter and was able to make decisions about her life that suited her, and not her family. She saw her family in a totally different light and was able to stop believing all the negativity they kept feeding her about herself. She is now able to put herself first and is very happy.

Getting rid of negative energy on a daily basis

I mention in this book that it is very easy to pick up negative energy from another person or building. This can attach itself to you and you may feel heavier and slightly depressed. If you work in a negative environment like a prison, it is essential that you do this on a daily basis.

One of the best ways of doing this is during your daily shower – turn the water to cold for a couple of minutes and ask that anything negative is blasted away from you and your aura (this is the area that surrounds your body and stops people getting too close to your personal area). Then ask to be filled with healing light.

It is a good idea to have a routine when coming home from work so you leave any negativity or stress behind. As a contractor I have always travelled for several hours a day to and from work. On a daily basis I would be stuck in traffic or see terrible accidents. Added to that I was working long hours and always under pressure because of deadlines. So I could have come home depressed, stressed and angry!! But as I walked down the garden path and would do the following:

- Ask that all negativity was removed from me
- I used to shake my hands as if I was shaking off the stress and the negativity
- I would play with my dogs who were greeting me with wagging tails and I would take on their love

So by the time I came in the back door I was as happy as Larry!!! So I suggest that you develop your own daily routine as it is not fair to bring all this negativity and stress home as it affects others in your household and will bring the energy down.

Also stop saying "I am stressed" as this keeps you in a cycle of stress. When you hear yourself saying this immediately stop yourself and replace with another statement. It could be something like "I am tired", "I a bit overwhelmed with everything at the moment but that is getting better" or "I need this little bit of stress to reach my deadline, but once that has gone, I will become distressed and happy again".

Meditation

The best way to de-stress yourself and keep yourself in tip top condition mentally, emotionally, spiritually and physical is to meditate daily. I don't mean that you have to sit in a room for hours on end chanting because none of us would do that – including me!

There are lots of different types of meditation around and you need to find the one that suits you. Can you sit and clear your mind for 10 minutes and not get distracted? If not then perhaps you need to listen to a cd or watch the flame of a candle.

If there are local meditation classes I would suggest that you join one so you can practice and see what it is all about. If you are a fan of youtube, why not watch and listen to their clips – I am all for making it as easy as possible!

If you are stressed at work a quick trip to the loo or your car for some meditation and deep breathing for 5 minutes will work wonders! Please do not be put off because you think it doesn't work or is weird. Throughout this book there are various exercises using meditation so this should get you familiar with the concept. If you are very tense the best form of meditation is to go through each muscle and tense it and then relax it.

Mindful meditation

This is a brilliant technique that you can use literally anywhere but especially when you are eating. You should be eating everything "mindfully" – that is in the present moment knowing exactly what you are doing!

Imagine the scene – you have gone to the bank and now you are the last in the queue and you are short of time. You can feel your stress levels rise and you starting tapping your fingers, breathing shallowly, and start becoming agitated – sound familiar?! Your boss is asking you to do something and **you are** panicking because you don't want to do it but you need time to form your answer so what do you do?

1. Breathe deeply in slowly for the count of 7 and then exhale for the count of 11. If you only have time to do this once before you have to give an answer, it should give you enough time to catch your breath and reply with a sensible answer. If you have time keep the breathing up for as long as you can

2. If you are in a queue or have time choose a spot in front of you – it could be a clock on a wall, the back of the person's head in front of you, a spot on a carpet or anything that takes your fancy. Using the breathing technique shown above, keep staring at this spot as you move up the queue in the bank or the supermarket. Keep repeating this until the task is completed and see how

different you feel! You will come out completely de-stressed and calm. This can also be used in a meeting or training course as you are completely 'with it' and can easily rejoin the discussion at will.

Using an ancient symbol – the Sri Yantra*

In my opinion this symbol has helped me reprogram myself positively more than any hypnosis cd. Look at the symbol and ask the Sri Yantra to connect you with everything your heart desires.

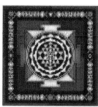

(if you would like a picture of a coloured Sri Yantra which is more powerful, please download one from the net).

What is the Sri Yantra? It is an ancient Hindu symbol which is used for meditation and is very powerful at activating your future desires. I would suggest that you use this symbol for at least 10 minutes per day and concentrate on keeping on track and losing weight.

Eliminating negatives with a positive

When a situation keeps going round in your mind it is very difficult to get rid of it. I was shown this exercise and it is excellent and can be used on anything from an emotion, to outside noise, to worrying about your job:

1. Pick a shape that you love and feel is peaceful – mine was a star
2. Pick a colour that you love and feel is peaceful – mine was amber
3. Pick a sound that you love and feel is peaceful – mine was OM
4. Pick a texture that you like and feel is peaceful – mine was satin
5. So think of the situation and then overlay the shape, then the colour, then the sound and then the texture.
6. Keep doing this until all negative emotions are released and you feel better

Grounding

When you are stressed or you experience a trauma, it is very easy to come 'out of your body'. This means that you can feel dizzy and 'not quite here on earth'. So it is very important to make sure that you are 'grounded' every day. Go outside and walk on grass in bare feet as often as you can and this really grounds you and connects you to the earth. The other routine I would recommend you do every day is:

- Stand with your feet on the ground
- Ask for roots to come down from the bottom of your feet into the earth and to wrap around beautiful crystals and metals. Feel yourself come back into your body and stand there for as long as you can
- Then ask for energy to come up the roots and go to every cell of your body
- Then ask for all negativity to go down the roots in the earth and be dissolved

Chapter 24:

CRYSTALS THAT HELP WITH WEIGHT LOSS AND THE METABOLISM

I absolutely adore crystals. I love their colours and their energy. I am particularly drawn to heart shape crystals When I was first married I used to collect porcelain figures and now I collect crystals and Buddhas. Crystal Buddhas are even better!

When you are holding a crystal remember that you receive energy in your left hand and it leaves your body through your right hand. So if the crystal is for encouraging energy hold it in your left hand. If the crystal is for releasing emotions or toxins hold it in the right hand.

You can place a crystal on any part of your body as well as holding it. You will gain added benefit with your weight loss and wellbeing if you hold a crystal over your heart, thyroid or third eye every day. You can buy a wand crystal and stroke it over a particular area or you could lie down and place a matrix of crystal around you while you relax. There are so many ways to receive the benefits of crystals.

Normally a crystal will choose you. You will be not be able to take your eyes off a crystal or if you hold your hand over a pile of crystals, the energy from one will bounce right up to your hand!

As with all the other techniques I talk about, it is essential to buy a good book on crystals because it will explain which crystals are used for which ailments and also how to keep them clean and programme them.

Most crystals need cleaning and the best way to do this, in most cases, is to put them in tepid water. If you can put them in the sun or the moonlight for a while that is even better. But you should look up the washing instructions for each crystal. This is particularly important when you bring a crystal home because it will have been handled by many negative people who will have transferred their negativity onto it.

When you have cleansed your crystal you need to programme it and get to know it. Hold it in your hand and feel the energy and the love. Thank the crystal for choosing you and send it love. The programming should relate to why you have purchased the crystal:

- I programme you to speed up my metabolism
- I programme you to help me lose weight
- I programme you to curb my appetite
- I programme you to improve my eyesight

If you don't want to spend a lot of money buying different crystals, you could buy one that really appeals to you and then programme it with all the areas that you want help with. So you could programme it to help you lose weight and lose water, curb your appetite and speed up your metabolism. This is most probably the best way to start off and it means that you can carry your crystal with you at all times.

Always thank your crystal when you have used it. Keep it out of direct sunlight and safe, perhaps in a nice velvet bag. If you drop it, apologise to it. Remember that the crystal has been living for a lot longer than you have. In other words treat it with respect.

Crystal Essences

One way of receiving the benefits of a crystal is to drink the crystal essence. To make the crystal essence, place a crystal in pure water and leave it for a couple of hours. Then take the crystal out and drink the water. The effects are amazing!

Crystals to help with the thyroid and metabolism

I am just listing crystals that help with the glandular system and metabolism. As the thyroid is the main gland responsible for metabolism, I outline mainly thyroid crystals. For crystals that help heal all other problems you can consult your newly purchased book. Chrysocolla is the crystal I use and carry around with me.

Chrysocolla Chrysocolla is an attractive blue-green crystal. This is a wonderful calming stone bringing inner peace and contentment. It is excellent on the emotional front, clearing guilt and negativity gently. It is used as a crystal for the throat chakra and therefore is excellent for the thyroid and increasing the metabolism.

Pyrolusite This crystal is silver in colour and made mostly from manganese. It is an excellent crystal for the eyesight and the metabolism. It also helps with mental and emotional clarity.

Sodalite Sodalite is a beautiful blue stone and is said to protect the user from negativity. It is used to assist in lowering blood pressure and balancing the metabolism and the entire glandular system. As it is a blue stone and related to the throat chakra it is good for communication.

Watermelon Tourmaline Tourmaline comes in many colours but Watermelon Tourmaline is particularly good for balancing the endocrine glands and the metabolism. It also balances the emotional system so it is excellent for emotional support. It also dispels fear and negativity.

Blue Calcite This is a beautiful pale blue crystal. It helps retain lessons learned and amplifies learning so it is particularly good for students. It also helps to calm in times of stress. It is also known to be used in healing of the throat, lungs, tonsillitis, thyroid, arthritis, joints and high blood pressure.

Lapis Lazuli Lapis Lazuli is a combination of Lazurite, Calcite and Pyrite and is the most beautiful shade of royal blue. Lapis Lazuli is said to enhance one's awareness, insight and intellect. It is also said to impart ancient knowledge and wisdom, bringing peacefulness and self-acceptance. Lapis Lazuli is said to help cure depression, insomnia, recurring fevers, vision and hearing problems, and disorders of the throat, lungs and immune system.

All blue crystals Because blue is the colour of the throat chakra, your thyroid will benefit from any blue crystal. Lie down and place the crystal over the thyroid in your throat area and relax.

Crystals for appetite control

We all need help controlling our appetite from time to time so carry one of these with you every day

Citrine	To level the appetite
Red Jasper	To control the appetite
Rhyolite	For inner strength, to encourage and support change
Tiger's Eye	Tiger's eye helps regulate eating habits
Increasing metabolism	Amazonite is the best crystal for this
Balancing blood sugar	Amethyst does this best
Water retention	Rose Quartz, Aquamarine and Jade are the best crystals for releasing water retention

Other Crystals that may be useful in your collection

My favourite wedding present is a large piece of rose quartz crystal as this signifies love and therefore makes an ideal present (and a different one at that!).

Rose Quartz	This crystal stands for love and is an amazing healing crystal
Amethyst	Amethyst is a beautiful purple stone that is an excellent all round healer
Clear Quartz	This is a must in everybody's collection as it can be used for meditation and healing

Section 7

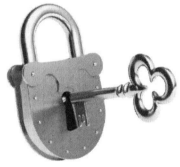

THE
'OOGIE GOOGIE'
STUFF

Chapter 25:
ANGELS AND GUIDES.
SOUL, INNER CHILD AND HIGHER SELF.
KARMA AND PAST LIVES.
WHAT ARE THEY AND HOW CAN THEY HELP YOU WITH YOUR WEIGHT LOSS NOW?

You have spirit guides and angels that guide you in your daily life and these can be harnessed to help you with your health and weight loss. You don't have to be religious to believe in these wonderful beings or karma. I certainly am not religious but have had experience of everything I write about in this section and I know it to be true.

This is why it is very important to connect to your inner self, which is a mixture of your higher self and soul so that all your problems are healed at the highest level and then they won't be recreated again. This is why you need to get to know 'all parts' of you so once again the problem is healed permanently – if you do not include your inner child or higher self in the healing it may want to hold onto the problem.

What is a Spirit Guide?

A spirit guide is a soul that has highly evolved to become a guide. It may have appeared in a human body on earth or it may have been working in the spirit world for all of its incarnation. For the purchase of this chapter I am also going to include different types of guides like goddesses such as Isis, ascended beings such as Jesus and other deities such as Genish and Lakshmi who are Indian gods. A spirit guide could also be a fairy or a goblin!

Before you incarnate, you and your spirit guides form a contract as to how long they are going to be with you and how they are going to help and advise you. You normally have one spirit guide that stays with you for all your time on earth. Mine is called White Arrow and he is a Native American Indian guide. Various spirit guides also come in and out of your life to help with problems such as health, money and relationships. But your guides are also learning and growing spiritually at the same time, so you are helping each other.

The spirit guide's job is to help and guide you through your human existence. Have you ever had a sudden inspirational idea and then wondered what made you think of it in the first place, especially as the idea actually works? Your guide impressed that idea to you via thoughts.

Some guides will show themselves to you when you connect with them. They may appear as monks or nuns, animals, Native American Indians, doctors or nurses – or they may choose to be invisible, or to show themselves as white light. They may give you a name or just pop in and out when you most need them. I once heard the saying "if you knew how many people walked with you, you would never feel alone" and this is so true. Because it is true you need to tune in with these guides so they can help you. As you have free will, they cannot help unless asked and only prompt you with ideas and opportunities – it is up to you to act on them.

When you become more experienced in working with your guides you can call in other guides to help with a particular issue. There are masses of books and information on the internet about spirit guides and if you are interested I would suggest that you do some research. This will enable you to always call in the right person for the job.

Why not ask your guides their names and really get to know them. Ask them to show themselves and find out whether you can see them clearly.

I work very closely with Merlin but will often ask to be sent a guide to help with a health or money issue. So start to call in your guides to help with healthy eating, releasing the excess water and weight and any emotional problems you may have. They will then guide you for hereon in.

Best guides for weight loss

Isis, Athena, Aphrodite, Kali, Lakshmi, Genish (as he removes obstacles) and Dana. I work with all these guides and they are a tremendous help and comfort.

My story
Spirit was sending me to various locations in the world to heal the land. I was confused about the next visit so I asked my guides. A week later I was reading a trashy magazine and saw an advert for a resort in the Bahamas that had many dolphins. I knew instantly that this was where I

should go to help heal these dolphins and I was lucky enough to spend a week with the beautiful creatures.

Before I went I was told that I would meet somebody who would show me where my next visit would be. The week went past and I met nobody, so I was getting worried – well, I shouldn't have been! I was sitting by the pool having my last coffee before leaving for my homeward journey when I spotted a lovely man having great fun with his young daughter in the pool. Surprisingly, they came and sat at my table in the lounge and we started to chat. It turned out that he had been stationed in the UK at an USAF base called Molesworth where I had lived for a short time when I was a child. What a coincidence, don't you think, as there are many USAF bases in the UK, but I knew at that moment that this man was going to tell me where my next trip was going to be! He and his wife then started to talk about their honeymoon. They had been to the Galapagos Islands – so I instantly knew I was being told to go there.

When I was on my weight loss journey I called in all the help I could get!! They would show me the healthy options and point me in the direction of the therapists that were right for me. I couldn't have done it without them!

You therefore need to be alert for signs from all sources and if you feel you are not getting help or any signs then ask again. Whatever you do, please do not think it has not worked and give up, as this will also restrict your communication and healing powers.

Why you have to look out for the signs

This is a joke but I think it describes the process very well!

A man was in a boat which capsized: he was starting to panic as he thought he was going to die. So he called out to God and asked for someone to be sent to help him. About an hour later the Royal Navy arrived and asked if would he like to be rescued but the man said no as God was saving him. Another hour passed and the Merchant Navy turned up and asked if he would like to be rescued and again he said no because God was rescuing him. A further hour later an air rescue helicopter turned up and asked if he would like to be rescued but for the third time the man said no - God was rescuing him. Then he drowned!

When he got up to heaven he said to God "Where were you? You were supposed to be rescuing me and I drowned". God replied "I sent the Royal Navy, Merchant Navy and an air rescue helicopter – what more did you want!"

The moral of this story is that you should look out for all signs, however unlikely – remember there is no such thing as coincidence!

My Story
My wonderful Native American Indian guide, White Arrow, appears to me with a beautiful wolf and I have a magnificent drawing of him and his wolf on my bedroom wall, so I go to sleep and wake up looking at their picture. Although I have other guides, White Arrow is always with me. He tells me he is learning as well and as I have chosen a complicated path where I seem to be continually studying, he must be learning a lot too! I can feel his strength and advice at all times.

What are Angels?

Angels have never incarnated and are messengers of God, depicted in most religions as beautiful white winged apparitions. We have a guardian angel and many other angels with us, guiding and helping us. Ask your angels their names and really get to know them so you can just think of their names and there they are.

So, as you would with your spirit guide, why not connect with your angels and ask how they are helping you. Angels have various jobs and are split into many groups – too many to go into here – but please read books on angels if you are interested.

On a day to day level they are amazing. If you lose your keys or you want a parking space, just ask them. I always find a parking space even when trying to park at Christmas, which is normally impossible! But remember, they can't help you unless you ask because of your free will but they are all there, hoping you are going to call on them because they like to be busy! Angels should always be called in when conducting a session for healing, help and guidance. So call in the weight loss angels now!

My story
My first recognition of angels was after my beloved Jack Russell, Oliver, died and I was inconsolable. I cried for days and lay on my bed

in a very depressed state, as he was quite simply the love of my life and I hadn't been ready for him to pass over. One day I felt the fluttering of wings and suddenly I felt an angel's wings wrapped round me and the angel lying down beside me, trying to comfort me and from that day I was totally convinced. I have also been aware of angels in difficult situations, especially in traffic, where you feel you are not going to stop or that somebody behind you is not going to stop and suddenly it is OK. There have been many reported sightings of angels transporting people out of the way of accidents, healing the sick and looking after the vulnerable.

Who are the best angels for weight loss?

Michael, Gabriel, Uriel, Maktiel, and Assiel (healer of water)

Dissolving dark energy
If you feel that you may have negative or dark energy, always call in the angels to dissolve it and replace it with white healing light. Ask that the angels stay as long as needed to ensure that you are healed.

Additional use of angels
If there has been a disaster or somebody has died or is ill, always ask for the appropriate angels to go to the area or the person or animal to give healing, love and comfort. Ask them to stay as long as necessary. If you can't find your keys or get a parking space your angels are happy to oblige!

What is a body elemental?
An elemental is a nature spirit and we are surrounded by these beautiful creatures. As we are spiritual, we also have an elemental that is called a body elemental. This body elemental helps us with our health and wellbeing – the problem is that it is trying to tell us what to do and because we don't know about them we totally ignore them. It is a good idea to connect with your body elemental and start to ask it what it needs to dramatically improve your health.

For example, before you eat anything ask your elemental if your body either needs it, wants it or if it is good for you. Ask your body elemental what exercise is the best for you and how often you should exercise. If you are stressed, ask your elemental why and what you can do to alleviate it.

My story

I got knocked over by a wave in Goa and it damaged my pelvis. My pelvis would tilt and the pain was unbelievable when it trapped my left leg and I would fall over. It stopped me from exercising and I was even frightened to walk down the stairs. I went to osteopaths and chiropractors but none could give me relief for more than ten minutes. Then I remembered my body elemental and asked her what was going on. She said that I had set up programmes of self-punishment as I felt I didn't deserve to be happy because of what I had done in past lives. So the constant pain was me punishing myself and I was suffering – and part of me was really pleased! So I worked to heal all these punishment issues and immediately my pelvis snapped back into place and has never gone out again.

What is your higher self?

Your higher self is the part of you that knows exactly what your incarnation plan is and what is best for you. Your higher self has been with you in previous lives and also knows your karma and what past lives need to be healed in this life. Ask your higher self to remove any of the emotions or weight that is nothing to do with you and that you have picked up from other people – this is quite common!

I would suggest that you call in your higher self and ask how your weight problem plays a part in your incarnation plan and how together you can lose the weight for good.

My story

I have been on a diet most of my life but have never been able to maintain a healthy body weight. I was in despair, so one day I called on my higher self to tell me why. What I was told was absolutely fascinating. My higher self told me I had died from starvation in previous incarnations and that my body held onto my weight as it was frightened I would starve. Also, when I was trying to lose weight I had cut my calories down to sometimes only 150 a day for seven years and my body was frightened I was going to do that again. When these issues were healed I started to lose weight.

A quick connection technique with your soul, spirit guides, angels, body elemental and higher self

Sit quietly, relax and breathe in and out very slowly so that you become calm and centered. When you breathe in ask that the white light surrounds and fills your body. This will make the connection easier as the white light will take you to the higher plane.

Ask for your spirit guide or whoever you wish to connect to, to come to you and ask that they give you a message or sign to confirm that they are there. You may go cold, see a symbol or get a message. You will get better at recognising the signs as you practice. But most of all have faith that they are with you and helping.

Then tell them what it is that you need help with. This could be anything from a health and weight issue to healing a row to finding a new job or clients. Sit quietly and see if you get any response but if you don't, don't worry, as the help may take some time to formulate in the universe. Look for signs that will indicate what is the best way for you to progress – it could be an advert in a magazine, an unexpected email popping into your inbox or a call from a friend who could help. Never disregard anything! At the end of the session, always thank whoever has been helping you.

This is also the way that you would do a quick connection to solve a particular issue.

Using meditation to connect to your soul, spirit guides, angels and body elemental

This meditation can be used to connect to your spirit guides, angels and body elemental. I would suggest that you use the short method to connect to your higher self.

At the beginning it is always best to connect to your guides, angels and your body elemental using the following meditation. Then when you are more practiced you will be able to call them in automatically when you need their help. Substitute 'spirit guide' with the name of the appropriate guide, angel and body elemental.

Meditation

Sit in a comfortable chair in a quiet space. I would suggest that you sit rather than lie down or you may fall asleep! Switch off your mobile phone and make sure you can't be disturbed by the land line ringing. You may wish to light a candle or burn some incense. Make sure that you are calm and relaxed and not angry or impatient. Start by breathing in white light and breathe out negative energy very slowly until you find yourself calm and relaxed and full of white light. Then start to breathe out white light as well as breathing it in. Ensure that your eyes are closed and that you are fully relaxed. Now you are ready to begin............

You find yourself in a meadow on a beautiful summer's day, surrounded by perfect flowers and animals. The sun is beating down on your face and you are happy. You sit on the grass and look at the beautiful flowers and delight in their magnificence. You ask the animals to come to you and they start to play and nuzzle you. This is as close to heaven that you have ever been! Know that you can stay here as long as you want and can return any time.

As you walk around the meadow you find a gate and you want to go through it. Open the gate and you find yourself in front of a huge wooden door in a turret. Open the door and go through into the turret and feel your excitement rising, as you know something wonderful is going to happen.

There is a spiral staircase going down, so walk slowly down the stairs until you get to the bottom and then find yourself in a desert which is full of unusual rocks. You decide to sit on a rock and look around as you are unsure where you are and what is going to happen. You suddenly get the urge to ask to see your spirit guide and you put the thought out into the universe.

Suddenly you see a figure in the distance coming to you slowly but it looks excited and it is waving at you. You know in your heart that this is your spirit guide and you start waving frantically back and you get up and start walking towards it. You embrace because you have known each other for millions of years and are happy to be back together. You have many questions, what name do you have, how are you, what are you doing - so you chat like you have never been apart. Ask all the questions that you want to, especially to do with your weight problem. Ask the guide what your purpose is in life and how to get started.

It is now time to part and you embrace again and your guide gives you a present for you to open when you return. You wave goodbye, saying you will meet again soon and walk back to the steps and you are walking lightly and you are very happy. You walk up the steps and at the top you go through the door and find the gate. You open the gate and walk back into the meadow. Here you sit down, surrounded by the animals and open your present. What is the gift and how is it going to help you in your life? Is it helping with weight loss or a money issue, is it for healing you, or is it for the planet? You are very grateful and you send thanks to your spirit guide for this gift.

Begin to wake up and come back to the room and stretch until you are fully awake.

When you are awake and back in the room, write down in your journal everything you have learned. What is your guide (angel, spirit guide etc) and what is its name? What present did it give you and what is it for? How is it going to help you in your day to day life? Decide that you are going to talk to it every day to build up a relationship so that you only have to think of it and it will be with you.

What is a soul?
If you believe you are a spiritual person in a human body you will already know that you have a soul. This is the part of you that travels from life to life with you and is programmed with past experiences so you can learn what you need to in this lifetime. It knows about all previous lives and also about future lives, what your incarnation plan is for this lifetime and how to bring it all together.

Humans and animals are here on earth to learn and grow. People find this concept difficult to understand and, if you are not on a spiritual path, I can see why. However, if we are not here to learn, why are we here? Surely not just to work, eat and sleep!

We chose this life before we came to earth and also what we are going to experience and learn. If your life seems hard and complicated that is because you have chosen it before you were born. All this learning is for our spiritual growth so eventually we do not return to earth but have another job somewhere in the universe. Mine is going to be sitting on a cloud with a harp!

So again develop relationship with your soul and heal why you decided to have a weight problem in this life. Your soul is waiting for you to ask for help!

All parts of you
As I have mentioned you are made up of many part as well as the ones I am talking about now. You may want to do some more research on these parts but it is important that they all play a part in your healing as they could be holding onto the missing key. These parts could be:

- Your physical body is surrounded by other bodies such as your etheric, emotional and mental
- You have archetypes which are called names like critical parent (inner critic) and your inner child
- You have personalities that have come from this or previous lives and could still be stuck in that time causing you problems

So when you ask to be healed be sure to include all these parts. Sometimes you will be directed to talk to a particular part as it has a story to tell before it will heal. Talk to them and find out what problems they are causing your life now. You could have a 3 yr old who was told she was bad, or an 8 yr old whose teacher told them that they would never amount to anything. Your inner child may not feel safe slim so wants to add more weight not less. Your emotional body may be traumatized and has you frozen and is stopping you moving forward.

What is karma and how does it affect your weight?

In Hinduism, karma is described as the total compilation of all a person's past lives and actions that result in the present condition of that person. Although this may be a bit of a mouthful and sound rather strange, it also translates into the more familiar expression, 'what goes round comes round'. Both relate to people's actions in the past that shape how they are now and in the future, and these actions can originate in this life or in a previous life.

Karma can relate to times in our life where we have caused others harm - either by our actions or words - or it can be from when others have caused us harm (for example, an attack, stealing money or bullying). That Karma then becomes part of our being and needs to be healed and released.

So if you constantly have money troubles, it could be because you stole money in previous lives (we all have!). This is why techniques like 'The Secret' or 'Cosmic Ordering' may not work for you because the karma has to be healed before money is allowed to flow to you.

It could be that you have decided to pay back your karma with your weight problem as this is causing you to suffer and punish yourself. Excess weight has often been referred to as "the heavy weight of karma".

My story
I was 12lb at birth and struggled all my life trying to lose weight and keep it off. When I started to look at karma I discovered that I had chosen this path as I felt I needed to punish myself and suffer for what I had done to others. As I had been an expert in water torture I had also decided to fill myself full of water as I had done this to many other people. When I healed and released all these past lives, the weight and water started to come off and I didn't feel I needed to be punished anymore.

Once you have learnt the lessons, realized that it was for your growth and you weren't going to do it again, your angels and guides will help you release it. Ask for their help daily until the karma around a particular issue is resolved.

Best angels and guides to help healing karma

The Lords of Karma, Archangel Michael and Gabriel and Merlin to work his magic!

What is dark and negative energy and how is it affecting you and your weight now?

If you are feeling low or depressed it is most probably due to the fact that you have picked up dark or negative energy. Because of the world situation and the turmoil, there is a massive amount of this energy and it can easily be picked up – especially if you drink, take drugs or are low and depressed. This unfortunately makes the situation much worse. There are also spirits that are waiting to attach to you and then can feed off you and this will increase your appetite. I don't want to scare you but certainly when you go into hospitals or grave yards there will be lost spirits waiting to attach to a physical body.

The best way for you to heal this is to ask the archangels and angels to come and heal and release this energy and then to fill yourself with white golden healing light. Ask that you are placed in a pink bubble and protected against such energy and attachments in the future.

Healing negative energy
The best ways to heal negative energy are:
- Ask the angels and guides to heal

- Hands on healing
- Crystals

Or book a session with me!

Curses

I don't want to frighten anybody but curses do exist and at the moment they are big business – some costing £5,000! Never, ever put a curse on somebody as it will immediately come back to you.

Curses can affect your weight and every other area of your life. It can be your own or it could be a curse that has come down your family line. If you feel you may be cursed please contact a qualified practitioner like myself to remove it. It is quite easy to do, so don't panic.

Somebody had put a curse on me many centuries ago and that is why I had filled up with water. It was a nun who I had had ducked during the witch trials and she wanted to get her own back – which she did very successfully I might add!

Vows and contracts

As most of us have had religious past lives and may have made contracts with people in this life, we need to tear these up. We should not be 'tied' to anybody or anything. Religious vows and can cause all sorts of problems as they can be of:
- Poverty
- Subservience
- Chastity
- Suffering

So these can not only give you 'lack' which in turn gives you a weight problem, but can make you broke as well. So call in all your guides and angels and any others that would like to come and help to tear up the contracts that no longer serve you and heal the damage.

How are past lives affecting your weight?

If you don't believe in reincarnation it may be an unfamiliar concept to accept but we have all lived before, some of us having had many lives and some having few. I seem to have had thousands. It is a very interesting subject, especially as it relates to how we are living now. So your weight problem could be because:
- You starved to death
- You died of malnutrition
- You had a past life where it was seen as prosperous to be overweight
- You died of thirst
- You were raped and don't want to be slim now
- You had a job that needed you to be big
- You had lack and scarcity or you caused other people to have it by stealing

My story
As you can imagine, I had all of these! I seemed to die of thirst on more desert islands than anybody I know. Apart from starving and dying of thirst, these are some of my other lives that have affected my weight:
- I had several lives in the South Pacific where it is considered beautiful to be large
- I also had several lives in Africa where I was force fed by a husband to make me bigger so that he appeared more prosperous
- I was a fat lady in a circus
- I was a sumo wrestler
- I had starved to death in a camp in Poland during the second world war

So call in your angels and guides and ask them to heal and release all the past lives that are causing your weight problem in this life. Ask them to program your subconscious so it knows that there is plenty now and that you are not going to die because of lack of food or water!

The power of prayer

There was a survey conducted in the States monitoring people who prayed every day asking for help with their weight problems and then compared them to people who didn't. Interestingly enough, the people who prayed lost more weight, so why not give it a go? Saying thanks or showing gratitude seems to have become unfashionable and people focus on what they don't have rather than what they have. So let's bring it back into fashion!

Pray every day and be thankful for what you have and the progress you make. We are inclined to take everything for granted and never give thanks. Go back to saying grace before a meal and if you eat animal protein, thanking the animal for giving its life to you. Remember that all illness or each problem is a lesson for you to learn, so be thankful for them - because of them you will spiritually grow.

If you believe that prayer will help you in your search for weight loss, go ahead and pray. You don't have to be religious but prayer is a way of asking for help. There is a marvellous website on prayers for weight loss www.beliefnet.com which lists masses of prayers that you can select from.

Chapter 26:

SPELLS FOR WEIGHT LOSS

I am absolutely fascinated by magic (white magic of course!). As I believe very heavily in negative karma, which you will have already read, there is no way that I would do a spell to hurt anybody or bring them misfortune. However, weight loss spells are a bit of fun and as I say many times in this book, it's worth a try! Also if you focus your attention on words, they do become real.

Have fun but remember that this is 'light-hearted'.

Simple weight loss spells

❖ What you need:
  • Clear quartz crystal
  • Green candle

Instructions: Choose a clear night, at least three days after the full moon (during the waning phase). If you can't do this spell outdoors, perform it near a window. Cast your circle in your usual manner. Light the candle and hold the crystal in your dominant hand. While watching the moon, recite these words:

> "Goddess within
> Goddess without
> Guide me to my goal
> Ease my hunger
> Soothe my spirit
> Strengthen my resolve
> As I will it, so mote it be".

Raise the crystal over your head and concentrate on all the negative aspects of losing weight (cravings, temptations, cheating etc). Draw these things out of you and put them into the crystal. If the candle is in a safe place, let it burn out. If you can't leave it, snuff it out. Carry the crystal with you (in a green pouch if you'd like).

From now on, every time you think about eating something (anything!) take out the crystal and ask yourself "do I need this or simply want it?"

This will remind you of your quest to lose weight and prompt you to think about what you are about to snack on.

❖ Stand in front of a mirror, put your hands on your stomach and chant these words with feeling:
> "Goddess hear my plead,
> Make me the weight I want to heed.
> This size is too big for me,
> A size (*size you want to be*) I want to be,
> So mote it be".

❖ Candle weight loss spell:
Meditate during the waning moon. Light a pink candle for self-love. Anoint it with the oil of your choice. Next light a brown candle, engrave the number of pounds you want to lose on it. Then visualize banishing the excess weight. Runes can also be carved on the candle if you wish and incense can be burned. Visualize the smoke taking the excess pounds away.

Take one white, one blue, and one yellow candle. Light them all in front of a mirror and say this chant:
> "Lighter thinner that I say
> Make me my right size this very day".

When you finish this chant, pour the wax from the candles into a small glass with a new wick in it. Repeat this day after day until your new candle is made. Burn your new candle until it or the wind puts the candle out. When you're feeling overweight again light the candle and let it put itself out.

More spells

These spells have come from an enormous selection on the internet so why not search for spells for your specific problems? Thank you to everyone who have written and published these spells. It is great fun and you are focusing all your attention on to your goal!

Section 8

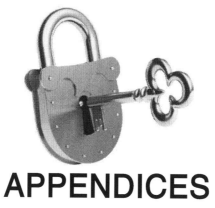

APPENDICES

Appendix I:
DIAGNOSTIC TOOLS

It is vital that anybody you see as a therapist can make an accurate diagnosis. I have had many therapies where the therapist worked from books, from answers to questions I gave and from their intuition and in every case their diagnosis was not accurate. Although they may have had years of experience, they were using what they 'felt' was right, not what was indeed right.

I would therefore like everybody to take responsibility for their life (and the life of anyone else they are looking after, which includes pets) and that means that they have to know exactly what to eat, what supplements or homeopathy to take, what physical treatments to have – even what moisturiser to wear.

To do this you need to have some form of diagnostic tool to use. There are two excellent diagnostic tools that I use which give an accurate analysis of the problem and an accurate course of treatment. These work on 'yes' or 'no' answers.

Remember that your body instinctively knows what is best for it and what it needs so the diagnostic tools are just tapping into this information.

I would recommend that you learn how to muscle test or use a crystal pendulum dowser and these are fully explained in this chapter. I dowse in Boots for shampoo and conditioner (much to everybody's amusement!) and I never have a treatment or buy a face cream without dowsing for it first. I even dowse on hotels in a country that I want to visit - in fact you can use it for everything.

When you read about dowsing and muscle testing you will think that I have gone totally mad (but you must be used to that now!). But when somebody has done a muscle test analysis on you, you can instantly feel the difference between 'yes' and 'no'. Then you become hooked and realise I am not as mad as you thought.

The best way of taking responsibility for your life and health is by having some form of diagnostic tool where you can either check someone else's results or you can choose your own therapies and herbs.

REMEMBER, IT IS PRACTICE, PRACTICE, PRACTICE
that gets results!
BOOK YOURSELF ON A COURSE NOW!

If you don't get any response to a question it will be because of the following:

- It can't be answered by a 'yes' or 'no' answer
- The question isn't clear enough and needs to be rephrased
- The answer is not known, as there is free will involved
- The question cannot be interpreted – for example you may ask "Will I be rich?" What is rich? You may need to ask "Will I earn £1,000 a week?"

Take the answer you get immediately and don't analyse it – this means you are putting your conscious mind on it and the answer could be what you want rather than what is going to happen.

Muscle testing

Muscle testing (also called Kinesiology) is where your arm muscle (usually your right arm muscle if you are right handed and your left arm muscle if you are left handed) is used to answer 'yes' or 'no' questions. You start by asking the body to identify your 'yes' or 'no' responses. Usually 'no' is a weak response (ie your arm will go weak when pressed down) and 'yes' is a strong response (ie your arm will not move when pressed down).

Normally you are in a standing position and you will be asked to raise your arm outstretched firmly to the side (but not locked) in line with your shoulder. I will then ask simple questions such as "Is Ann your name?" and when I press lightly on your arm it will go down very quickly (unless your name is Ann, of course!). Then I will ask "Is your name 'your name'?" and when I press on your arm it will remain in line with your shoulder.

You must NEVER try to force an outcome – let the arm give you the answer.

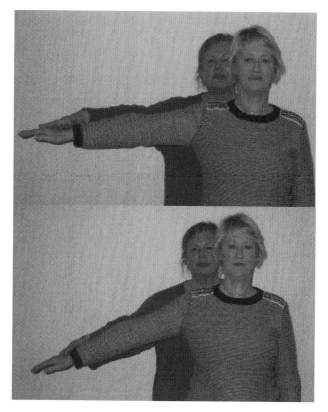

An example of you muscle testing somebody else:

1. Stand behind your friend and ask them to hold their right arm out to the side of the body. If they are left handed you should be using their left arm.
2. The arm should be firm but not locked
3. With your finger pressing very lightly on their forearm ask "Please give me a 'yes' answer". Note whether the arm moves freely or stays the same. Whichever one it is will become your 'yes'.
4. Repeat Point 3 but ask for a 'no' answer – it should be the opposite response to 'yes'.
5. Then start asking questions that can be answered with a 'yes' or 'no' response:
   i. Is xxxxx deficient in Vitamin B
   ii. Put a bowl of sugar in the friend's left hand and then ask: Does xxxxx have an intolerance to sugar?"
   iii. "Does xxxxx want to lose weight?"

Do have fun with these, they are just a taster for you to try but remember that muscle testing is an amazing diagnostic tool. Some therapists will test you using other muscles of the body.

Your friend's arm may get a little stiff or sore. If this happens ask him/her to release their arm and do some gentle shoulder lifting exercises before resuming the pose.

Personal muscle testing
Wouldn't it be handy if you could muscle test on yourself. You could get clear and concise information on yourself in any situation - the good news is that you can!

I have two ways of doing this:

1. Programming of hands:
I programmed my hands to give 'yes' or 'no' answers. I sat with both hands at right angles to my wrists. I then said "Please show me a strong reaction as to which hand would like to be 'yes'" and one hand will move downwards – this will then become your 'yes' hand (mine is my right hand). Your hand may not move but you may get tingling or it may go hot or cold but there will be a sign. If nothing happens, speak again until you get a reaction.

Then repeat the operation for 'no' – this should be your other hand! It is like a cross between muscle testing and dowsing and it means that even if I am in the car I can ask questions about myself, for example, should I take a particular road to avoid the traffic.

'Don't know' or 'Unsure' mean that neither hand will move.

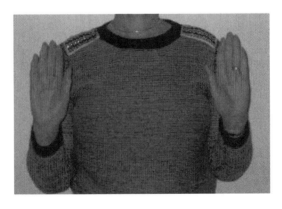

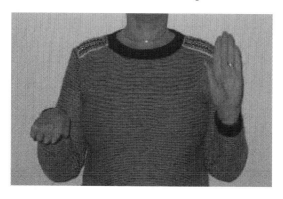

2. Self-muscle testing using fingers

It is amazing how your body reacts to suggestion and this particular exercise never ceases to amaze me. I put my first finger on top of my thumb nail. The way you programme your two fingers is by (a) keeping them together and (b) pulling them apart.

Ask your fingers to give you a 'yes' answer. Your fingers will either be tight together or your first finger will slip off your thumb. My 'yes' is that my thumb and finger stay tightly locked together (and I mean tightly). When I ask for 'no', my finger immediately separates from and falls off my thumb – its still amazes me even to today.

You can also surrogately use muscle testing. "Should little Johnny have this vaccine?" is a very useful one.

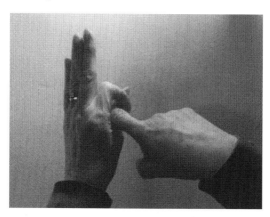

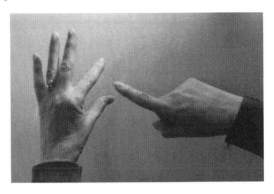

3. Programming of the body

You use your body in much the same way as your hands to programme it. I asked my body "Please show me my 'yes' and my body swung forward. I then repeated the operation for 'no' and my body swung backwards. Make sure you don't fall over when you do this!

Using a Crystal Dowsing Pendulum

Dowsing with a crystal pendulum is a good diagnostic tool and I use this method every day in my life.

Once again dowsing works on the energy that is surrounding you and will answer 'yes' or 'no' questions. It can also be used to find lost items and can be quicker than muscle testing for identifying other areas, such as which colour you should wear or the Bach Flower Remedy you should take. I would suggest that you buy a pendulum and start practising (remember that practise with all therapies is essential) as you will come to rely on it wholeheartedly.

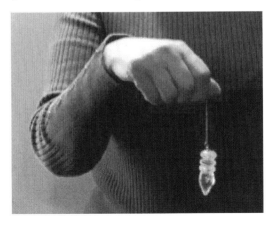

1. Buy a clear quartz (*) pendulum, wash it in warmish water and dry it lovingly. Thank the dowser for coming to help you and as you are holding this lovely clear quartz dowser ask it to help you get the best results from your dowsing together (this is programming it). Keep it safe and in a special container, perhaps a velvet bag.

2. Holding the chain on the pendulum swing it slightly backwards and forwards and ask it to show you its 'yes' response. Note which way the pendulum starts to turn. This may seem slow but this is quite normal. Also you may feel that you are forcing it and this is quite normal as well! My 'yes' is a right (clockwise) circle.

3. Repeat point 2 and ask for your 'no' response – mine is a left (anticlockwise circle).

4. Repeat point 2 and ask for a 'not sure' response. Mine is a diagonal swing from a north-west direction to a south-west direction.

5. Repeat points 2-4 to double check your answers.

6. Get dowsing!

7. Always thank your dowser for its help after you have finished a session and pop it back into it container.

8. Remember to wash and reprogram it frequently.

9. Always start a dowsing session with a clear mind and set the intention that the dowsing will be for everybody's highest good. It is essential that you don't have any preconception of the real answer, or of the answer that the person wants so the less you know the better!

10. Don't keep asking the same question otherwise your dowser will get fed up and start giving conflicting information.

11. If you feel you are getting wrong answers have a rest and a glass of water and return to the dowsing when you feel fresher.

12. Remember that you need to practice, practice, practice and trust totally in the information that you are being given.

   ❖ You may wish to purchase another crystal to use as a pendulum. Choose one that catches your eye or jumps out at you. Some people use wood, brass or gold/silver as some therapists recommend them for certain tasks. I am more of a believer in one pendulum as I feel you create a relationship with it.

Intuition

Everybody has this but most people totally disregard what they get. How many times have you heard someone say that they had a 'gut feeling' – that is intuition. When the phone goes and you know who it is before you pick it up – that is intuition. You need to start listening to your inner dowser or muscle tester and when something comes up don't try and reason with what you get, just accept it and write it down.

Meditation helps with listening to your intuition because you are quiet and are listening. When you are busy and rushing around there is no time or space for anything to come in.

When you start trusting you will become more and more intuitive and remember that this takes practise too.

Appendix II:
EMOTIONAL FREEDOM TECHNIQUE™ SHORT GUIDE

Scan in the following two sheets which are the EFT™ Short Guide. You could print it double sided and perhaps A5 and you could even laminate it. You can carry it around with you so you can tap at any time and you won't forget the points.

EFT™ SHORT GUIDE

ALL TAPPING POINTS

TOP	Top of Head
EB	Beginning of Eyebrow
SE	Side of the Eye
UE	Under the Eye
UN	Under the Nose
CH	Crease of the Chin
CB	Beginning of the Collarbone
UA	Under the Arm
IW	Inside the Wrist
TH	Thumb
IF	Index Finger
MF	Middle Finger
LF	Little Finger
KC	Karate Chop

THE FULL TAPPING SEQUENCE

STEP 1

TUNING INTO THE PROBLEM Tune into the problem and then give it a number out of 10 which is the intensity (0 is no intensity, 10 is acute density). For example, the problem is "I cannot lose weight", the intensity being 10 out of 10. This number will go down during the session and when it gets to 0 this particular problem has been cleared. At the end of the Full Tapping Sequence it is essential that you rate your intensity number to ensure that it has gone down. If it hasn't you are not connected to the correct emotion or the words are not describing the emotion in the correct way – change your wording, speak louder and persevere.

STEP 2

THE SET UP The Setup consists of a phrase or word that describes your problem, such as "I can't lose weight". You repeat this phrase three times whilst tapping on the KC point (Karate Chop): "Even though I have this …. (insert your problem or uncomfortable/distressing feeling), I deeply and completely accept myself" (or other suitable positive phrase).

STEP 3

THE TAPPING SEQUENCE AND REMINDER PHRASE - Using two or three finger tips, tap at least seven times firmly on each of the Tapping Points whilst repeating a Reminder Phrase. The Reminder Phrase is a cut down version of the Setup Statement like weight; hate my job, no money – or whatever feels right to you.

Tapping Points: EB : SE : UE: UN : Ch : CB : UA : Th : IF : MF : LF : KC

STEP 4

THE 9 GAMUT PROCEDURE This step helps release the emotions very quickly but does seem a little strange! Keeping your head still, continuously tap on the Gamut Point (which is in the gap on the back of your hand between the knuckles of your ring

360

finger and little finger) whilst performing the following nine actions (there is no need to repeat the reminder phrase on this part):

1	Eyes closed	2	Eyes open
3	Eyes look hard down right	4	Eyes look hard down left
5	Roll eyes in a huge circle	6	Roll eyes in the other direction
7	Hum Happy Birthday for two seconds	8	Count from 1 to 5
9	Hum Happy Birthday for two second		

STEP 5
THE SUBSEQUENT TAPPING SEQUENCES – Repeat Step 3 until you reach the KC point. This round is now complete. If the intensity hasn't gone to 0, keep repeating Step 5 until it gets below an intensity of 4. You can now start from Step 1 again and this time amend your Set Up Phrase to "Even though I **STILL** have this problem, I ...."

ASPECTS OF A PROBLEM - If you have a problem it is bound to be many aspects. You may be frightened of snakes but there could be lots of aspects to this, for example, the way the snake moves, how it might kill you, how its tongue pokes out.

SURROGATE TAPPING - You can surrogately tap on a friend, member of your family or a pet using all the different tapping sequences. So instead of tuning into your problem you tune into their problem and give it an intensity rating out of 10. The only difference is that the set up statement will be "Even though 'insert name of the person here' has this problem...."

MORE ADVANCED TAPPING ROUTINES
When you are more experienced you most probably will not need to use the Full Tapping Sequence as there are a variety of quick short forms. However, if the intensity number does not reduce, always return to the full tapping routine.
- You can use the inner wrist point instead of tapping on all the finger points
- You can exclude the setup statement and gamut point using the following points and saying different statements at each point:

TOP	I can't lose weight
UN	I eat because I am bored
CH	It is too difficult to lose weight
EB	I am obsessed with food
CB	I am frightened to lose weight
SE	I will feel deprived if I diet
UA	I will fail
UE	I am not safe if I lose weight

Just think of the problem and keep tapping the KC point until you feel something release

TAPPING IN THE POSITIVE - When your problem has reached the intensity rating of 0, you will want to tap in the positive, so use the tapping points specified using a positive statement such as 'I will not feel deprived if I diet'.

Appendix III:
THE BEST WEIGHT LOSS TIPS

These are some of my weight loss tips to help you on your way!

Practical weight loss tips

- Keep a food journal of everything you eat, your emotions and how you feel so you can track when you overeat, comfort eat, cheat or have emotional problems
- Tot up the calories to make sure you are on the right track and make sure you over estimate! Also keep track of sugars and fats as well
- Always check the calories on processed foods – sandwiches can be nearly 1000 calories!
- Don't go shopping hungry
- Clear all negative food from your cupboards and freezer
- Always have prepared snacks so you don't reach for the chocolate
- Make your own sandwiches – you don't need all that butter as well as mayo!
- Watch the olive oil – it may be healthy but it is calorific!
- When you go out to eat cut out the bread and butter and have one course!
- Swop to low calorie mayo and salad cream and use in sandwiches and jacket spuds
- Try not combining protein with carbohydrates – not only will your food digest quicker but you will cut your calories
- Make sure you have 5 vegetables and 1 fruit and not 5 fruit – vegetables contain more vitamins and minerals and are less calorific
- Don't eat carbohydrates after 6.30
- Eat a little in the evening – perhaps some vegetable soup – so you are not going to bed full
- Swop sugar for Stevia which is a healthy herb and balances your blood sugar level as well!
- Always grill and steam – do not use your microwave as that kills food and it has no goodness left. Even though the fashion is not to

fry please don't – even olive oil is toxic and it still adds a lot of calories
- Have a diet buddy who you can ring or join a club for a social weighing and chat
- Be sponsored to lose weight – that works!
- Use an aromatherapy oil to help release weight, appetite and water retention
- Use a crystal to help with weight loss
- Take responsibility for your weight and read up about new techniques, supplements, herbs etc
- Eat off a blue or purple plate – this is an appetite suppressant!
- Eat off a smaller plate – but make sure you only eat off one!
- When you eat fruit always make sure you eat a couple of nuts with it as this stops it being stored as fat!
- If you put on a couple of pounds at the weekend work out how you are going to get them off quickly as they remain as water in your body for 48 hours. Cut down, fast or just eat vegetables until the pounds have gone!
- Work out how you are going to use your eating plan for life – do you fast on a Monday or just eat juices? Do you eat what you want on a Sunday but watch it the rest of the week – what works best for you?
- Only eat when you are hungry and stop BEFORE you are full as it takes a while for the FULL message to get to the brain
- Just because your mother told you you had to clear your plate it doesn't mean that you have to! You are an adult now!
- Just because your mother made you feel guilty for leaving something on your plate because of the starving children in African doesn't mean that you have to eat anything
- Always leave something on your plate
- Eat slowly and chew every mouthful thoroughly before swallowing!
- Sit at a table to eat a meal and not on the go or standing up
- Make an occasion out of a meal with setting the table nicely
- Award yourself a non food treat every day
- Award a bigger treat every week or when you have reached a milestone
- Put your knife and fork down between each mouthful
- Chew every mouthful at least 20 times

- Don't drink alcohol as this retains water and wastes calories!!
- Eat one square of chocolate not the bar! I can help you with this so tweet me!
- If you want something to eat wait 15 minutes and if you still want it have it!
- Use a free weight loss subliminal software messenger on your computer
- Have a clay body wrap – they really do work! Make sure you have an experienced wrapper who has been doing it for at least 6 months
- Don't eat the kid's leftovers!
- Buy good kitchen scales so you can educate yourself what 2 ozs of cheese really looks like!
- Accept who you are and that being slim might not make you as happy as you think it will!
- Ask your body what it wants, become friends with it and treat it like your best friend!
- Love yourself and love your body and accept yourself – the struggle will make it worse
- Eat low GI foods for slow release and weight loss
- Write down short term and long term goals and stick to them!
- Don't beat yourself up and be nice to yourself – you wouldn't treat a friend like this!
- Cut back on salt as this can retain water
- If you crave crisps your adrenals need help so investigate supplements on the internet
- If you crave sweet things your hormones may be out of balance so investigate supplements on the internet
- Make small changes that will last a lifetime – like walking, watching what you are eating and drinking!
- Decide this is the last time you are going to lose weight and you are going to keep it off for life!
- Every 10 years your metabolism slows down by 10% so you need to adjust your intake accordingly
- Always eat fruit in between meals as it will interfere with digestion if eaten after a meal
- Add healthy fats to your diet like nuts, seeds, and omega 3
- Be clear on what your motivations are for losing weight – do it for yourself and not for anybody else!

- Work out what triggers your eating so I can clear it for you!
- Be aware of all or nothing eating and work out why you are doing it
- Read food labels carefully for added fats, sugar and salt
- Practise saying NO – if people are offended that is their problem
- Always watch your portion size – remember it should never be bigger than you can fit in the palm of your hand!
- Believe in yourself and that you can do this – let this become your daily mantra!
- Don't buy anything you crave like peanuts or chocolate as you won't be able to resist them!
- Don't leave food out like chocolate as this is temptation but eat in moderation
- Put a fat picture of yourself on the fridge door – remember 'fridge pickers wear big knickers!' or put a slim picture of yourself on the fridge – whichever way will motivate you
- If you don't know how much you are eating, lay a whole day of food out on the table and take a photo of it – you may be surprised how much you are eating! Then put it on facebook!
- Ensure you are having a slightly alkaline diet as the fat can't come out of the cells if your body is acid
- Get plenty of sleep especially if you are a child as this is a cause of weight gain!
- Eat before a night out or a party so you don't overeat on fattening things
- Ask for food without salad dressing or fattening sauces
- Protein keeps you fuller longer so eat some at every meal
- Do not starve yourself as this will slow down your metabolism
- Use a technique like EFT to reduce your 'set point' to a lower level if you are reached a weight plateau
- Eat lots of oily fish every week
- Do set realistic goals that you can stick to and don't become a burden
- Don't keep getting onto the scales as this can depress you – you will know you are losing weight by your clothes
- Don't be desperate as this will stop you losing weight as it slows down your psychic connection
- Moderation in everything – just because the diet says unlimited meat it doesn't mean you can eat a whole chicken!

- Breathe deeply before you are about to cheat or eat something – this will change your feelings and you most probably won't want it anymore
- Make sure you are taking supplements because you need the full amount of vitamins and supplements to lose weight
- Don't put butter on bread or potatoes – you really don't need it and it is so calorific!
- Buy small of everything – spuds, eggs, bananas – this will really cut down on the calories
- Don't overeat on holiday – you should be eating lots of fish and salad!
- Remember this saying – a minute on the lips, a lifetime on the hips!
- Don't worry if your weight doesn't match what the predetermined scale says – when I was almost skeletal on these scales I showed up as obese!
- Don't get obsessed by BMI measurements – go by how you feel and how your clothes feel
- If you want to have a biscuit have a jaffa cake – they are only 45 calories!
- Beware of healthy eating bars – they are usually calorific, full of fats and sugars and artificial sweeteners
- Don't use artificial sweeteners as they can cause weight gain and are really bad for your body!
- Olive oil may be good for you but it is so calorific – have a couple of olives a day and take Omega 3's! It is not just the oil that makes the Mediterranean diet good for you – that is the fish, vegetables and fruit!
- Cut out a picture of the body you would like and stick your head on it and pin it somewhere where you look at it all the time – this is programming your subconscious to the new you!
- Have a diet buddy who you can ring or join a club for a social weighing and chat
- Be sponsored to lose weight – that works!
- Join a group such as Weight Watchers or Slimming World
- Eat mindfully so you know what you are eating and enjoy every mouthful
- Remember that you have WILLPOWER – remember to use it!!!
- Use an aromatherapy oil to help release weight, appetite and water retention

- Use a crystal to help with weight loss
- Take responsibility for your weight and read up about new techniques, supplements, herbs etc
- Just because your mother told you you had to clear your plate it doesn't mean that you have to! You are an adult now!
- Eat slowly and chew every mouthful thoroughly before swallowing!
- Sit at a table to eat a meal and not on the go or standing up
- Make an occasion out of a meal with setting the table nicely
- Award yourself a non food treat every day
- Award a bigger treat every week or when you have reached a milestone
- Put your knife and fork down between each mouthful
- Eat one square of chocolate not the bar! I can help you with this so tweet me!
- If you want something to eat wait 15 minutes and if you still want it have it!
- Use a free weight loss subliminal software messenger on your computer
- Have a clay body wrap – they really do work! Make sure you have an experienced wrapper who has been doing it for at least 6 months
- Buy good kitchen scales so you can educate yourself what 2 ozs of cheese really looks like!
- Accept who you are and that being slim might not make you as happy as you think it will!
- Ask your body what it wants, become friends with it and treat it like your best friend!
- Love yourself and love your body and accept yourself – the struggle will make it worse
- Write down short term and long term goals and stick to them!
- Don't beat yourself up and be nice to yourself – you wouldn't treat a friend like this!
- Make small changes that will last a lifetime – like walking, watching what you are eating and drinking!
- Decide this is the last time you are going to lose weight and you are going to keep it off for life!
- Every 10 years your metabolism slows down by 10% so you need to adjust your intake accordingly

- Be clear on what your motivations are for losing weight – do it for yourself and not for anybody else!
- Work out what triggers your eating so I can clear it for you!
- Be aware of all or nothing eating and work out why you are doing it
- Believe in yourself and that you can do this – let this become your daily mantra!
- Don't buy anything you crave like peanuts or chocolate as you won't be able to resist them
- Get plenty of sleep especially if you are a child as this is a cause of weight gain!
- Eat before a night out or a party so you don't overeat on fattening things
- Do not starve yourself as this will slow down your metabolism
- Do set realistic goals that you can stick to and don't become a burden
- Moderation in everything – just because the diet says unlimited meat it doesn't mean you can eat a whole chicken!
- Learn how to do self-hypnosis so you can reprogram your subconscious!
- Use affirmations every day

Weight Loss tips for Food

- Plan your weeks food and write a menu and only shop for that food
- Eat a little in the evening – perhaps some vegetable soup – so you are not going to bed full
- Swop sugar for Stevia which is a healthy herb and balances your blood sugar level as well!
- Always grill and steam – do not use your microwave as that kills food and it has no goodness left
- Eat healthy fat and don't forget that they are now saying that eggs are good for you!
- Cut out all fizzy drinks – they are really bad for you and will retain water and make you hungry
- Cut out all biscuits, cakes, crisps and anything else with trans-fats in it – why not make your own low calorie versions?

- When you eat fruit always make sure you eat a couple of nuts with it as this stops it being stored as fat!
- Drink plenty of water and drink a glass 30 minutes before a meal which does fill you up! Sip the water otherwise it will go straight through you! Avoid fizzy water as this can retain water
- Think about what you can add to your diet not take away – for example different vegetables, sugar free jelly or miso
- Don't eat the kid's leftovers!
- Eat low GI foods for slow release and weight loss
- Cut back on salt as this can retain water
- If you crave crisps your adrenals need help so investigate supplements on the internet
- If you crave sweet things your hormones may be out of balance so investigate supplements on the internet
- Alcohol strips out all the vitamins and minerals out of your body – another reason to stop!
- Always eat fruit in between meals as it will interfere with digestion if eaten after a meal
- Add healthy fats to your diet like nuts, seeds, and omega 3
- Read food labels carefully for added fats and salt
- Always watch your portion size – remember it should never be bigger than you can fit in the palm of your hand
- Don't leave food out like chocolate as this is temptation but eat in moderation
- Ask for food without salad dressing or fattening sauces
- Protein keeps you fuller longer so eat some at every meal
- Eat lots of oily fish every week
- Don't put butter on bread or potatoes – you really don't need it and it is so calorific!
- Beware of healthy eating bars – they are usually calorific, full of fats and sugars and artificial sweeteners
- Don't use artificial sweeteners as they can cause weight gain and are really bad for your body!
- Add salad and vegetables to everything you eat! Pasta - put vegetables with the sauce and have a side salad; add a salad to a pizza; add salad to a sandwich; always have chopped up salad for snacking; add a salad to a jacket spud

- Did you know that doctors are now saying that eating 1200 calories a day is really good for you as it reduces inflammation and kicks in the longevity gene!
- Doctors are now also saying that fasting is good for you – why don't you try it for one or two days a week?
- Use EFT ᵗᵐ to change your beliefs so that you think Kale is better than chocolate – yes it can be done!

Weight loss tips for supplements

- Use an appetite suppressant like Hoodia to help the hunger plan
- Stimulate your metabolism by using chili, black pepper and herbs
- Take chromium to help with cravings
- Cinnamon can help balance your blood sugar level
- Make sure you are taking supplements because you need the full amount of vitamins and supplements to lose weight
- Investigate HCG homeopathy drops for quick weight loss that also help your endocrine system
- Vitamin D is needed in large quantities for weight loss
- If you suffer with SAD investigate St John's Wort to stop you putting on weight in the winter
- Chubby cheeks? It could be the alcohol you are drinking causing water retention – cut down!
- Hefty thighs? Could be your hormones are to blame. Make sure you eat to balance your hormones and cut out alcohol. Could also be genes past down so blame your mother!
- Love handles? You are not handling insulin well. Cut down on sugar and eat plenty of protein with vegs. Take a multi vitamin and take chromium
- Bingo wings? You are estrogen dependant so get your hormones checked. Could also be environmental toxins. Make sure you do plenty of exercise to release toxins
- Wobbly tummy? You could be stressed and have too much of the hormone cortisol. Eat well and make sure you are getting your nutrients. Try to calm down!
- Chunky Calves? You could be tired so up your sleep. It could be water retention so try a diuretic
- Bra strap bulge? You are not handling carbohydrates properly. Cut out grains and carbs for at least 3 months and then introduce slowly but not excessively

Exercise weight loss tips

- Do deep breathing exercises as this will increase oxygen and increase your metabolism
- Fit into your day 1 hour of exercise and make it fun so you will stick to it – put on your favourite cd and dance, walk your dog, make house work exercise!
- Ensure that you are getting the vitamins and minerals you need so supplement if necessary
- Walk when you can and leave the car at home!
- Don't waste a moment for exercise – clench your bottom muscles in the supermarket queue or while you are waiting for the kettle to boil; use arm weights during your favourite soap
- Don't forget to exercise your face because that will really show when you lose weight!
- Find out the best exercise for your body shape
- Try to exercise every day even if it is running upstairs
- Don't take the lift just run up the stairs!
- Do lots of different exercises – yoga, pilates, gym, callenetics, high cardio – variety is good!

Appendix IV:
A SELECTION OF WEIGHT LOSS AFFIRMATIONS

- I love, value and respect myself
- I deserve to have the body I want
- I can say NO to everything I don't want to do and that includes eating or drinking
- Every day in every way I am getting slimmer and slimmer
- Every day in every way I am getting fitter and fitter
- I am relaxed, peaceful and calm when I eat
- I eat only when I am hungry
- I stop eating before I am full
- I feel good about myself
- My body naturally sheds unneeded fat
- I have full ability to control my weight
- My appetite is easily satisfied with a small amount of food
- My body gets all the nutrients it needs
- My body is dissolving excess fat for it no longer needs it
- I am strong, fit and healthy
- My appetite for fattening and sweet foods has dissolved
- I am not tempted by fattening food
- I am not tempted by other people
- I see myself as slender, fit, and trim
- I am easily satisfied with my small meals
- I have tremendous self-control to stay to my diet
- I have a strong urge to eat only health-giving and nutritious foods
- I take good care of my body
- I love and accept myself
- I do a healthy amount of exercise regularly
- I like and love myself
- I have perfect control of my weight
- I refuse junk food and I eat healthy foods only
- I love nutritious foods
- I am attaining and maintaining my ideal weight

- I am willing to change
- I give myself permission to lose weight
- I deserve to lose weight
- Everything I eat encourages weight loss
- I have the power to change my life
- I eat only what I need
- I am committed to my goals
- I eat foods that support my new weight
- I think, act and eat like a slim person
- I love my body and treat it with respect
- I leave food on my plate as I am always full
- I have tremendous will power
- I choose to eat healthy foods and I enjoy salads, fruits and vegetables
- I choose to wear clothes that show of my leaner body
- Because I love myself I eat only what I need
- I choose only food that gives me energy
- It is easy for me to stop and relax before I eat
- I am losing weight now
- I am worthy of love and attention
- I know I deserve a lean and healthy body
- I love the way my lean body feels
- I love myself now and I will love my body as I show it the respect it deserves
- Just because it is meal time, doesn't mean I need to eat
- I celebrate my own power to make choices around food
- I know the consequences of overeating and it is easy to make the right choices
- It is easy for me to change my eating habits
- My body is becoming stronger and more attractive every day
- I am attractive, I am sexy and I am beautiful
- I have a great figure and I am proud when others notice my new body
- I enjoy waiting for dinner, because I enjoy it more when I wait
- I chew slowly and eat mindfully
- I always decide bite after bite if I really want more
- I enjoy my new eating habits, they support me.
- Every day my relationship with food becomes healthier

- I am learning and using the mental, emotional, and spiritual skills for success
- I am willing to change!
- It's exciting to discover my unique food and exercise system for weight loss
- I am delighted to be the ideal weight for me
- I choose to embrace thoughts of confidence in my ability to make positive changes in my life
- It feels good to move my body. Exercise is fun!
- I use deep breathing to help me relax and handle stress
- I deserve to be at my ideal weight
- It is safe for me to lose weight
- It is safe for me to be slim and attractive
- My metabolism is excellent
- I easily achieve all my goals and dreams
- I am totally confident
- I have a high self esteem
- I have the extraordinary ability to accomplish everything I choose and want
- I am committed, determined and passionate about what I do
- I am a very focussed and persistent
- I have tremendous energy and focus for achieving all my goals
- I am a master at what I do
- I feel happy and at peace with myself
- I meditate daily and stay in constant sync with the vibration of abundance and success
- My inner vision is always clear and focused.
- Today, I will concentrate on taking one step forward, however small
- I focus my power and I change my life
- I can accomplish anything I set my mind to
- Everything I touch is a success
- I am confident, competent and calm
- I am persistent, I persevere and I win!
- I am organised and disciplined
- I expect everything to go right and it does!
- I can lose weight and keep it off with ease

Appendix V:
RECOMMENDED READING LIST

The books listed below are all in my collection. I have either talked about them in this book or they are about subjects very close to my heart. I recommend that you read as many as possible.

All these books are available on Amazon or on the internet, so I haven't added the ISBN number.

The Medical Medium	Antony Williams
Your thyroid problem solved	Sandra Cabot
Wilson's Syndrome	Dr Wilson
The Tibetan Art of Positive Thinking	Christopher Handsard
Ask and it is given	Ester and Jerry Hicks
Fat Land – How Americans became the fattest people in the world	Greg Critser
The Slow Poisoning of America	John and Michelle Erb
I can Make you Slim (+ CD) *I can Make you Happy (+ CD)* *I can Make you Confident (+ CD)* *Gastric Band CD*	Paul McKenna
We are the Angels (about Karma)	Diane Stein
All Women are Healers	Diane Stein
Radical Forgiveness	Colin Tipping
The book of Miracles	Kenneth Woodward
The hidden messages in water	Masaru Emoto

The New Psycho-Cybernetics	Maxwell Maltz
The Wrinkle Cure	N V Perricone
7 Secrets to Beauty, Health and Longevity	N V Perricone
The Perricone Weight-Loss Diet	N V Perricone
Dr Nicholas Perricone's Programme	N V Perricone
Total Health	Joseph Mercola
Sweet deception	Joseph Mercola
Eat Right for your Type	Dr. Peter J. D'Adamo
Metabolic typing	William Linz
In Balance for Life (ph)	Alex Guerrero
Hormone Solution	Thierry Hertoghe
The liver cleansing diet	Sandra Cabot
Fats that heal, fats that kill	Udo Erasmus
Jumpstart your metabolism	Pam Grout
PACE exercise	Al Sears
Mastering Leptin	Byron Richards and Mary Richards
Turn off your fat genes	Dean Ornish and Neal D. Barnard
Miracle Doctors	Jon Barron
Shaman Healer Sage	Alberto Villodlo
Soul Wisdom	Dr Zhi Gang Sha

Appendix VI:
RECOMMENDED INTERNET SITES

Wilson's Syndrome	www.wtsmed.com
Joe Mercola	www.mercola.com
Al Sears	www.alsearsmd.com
Cranial Sacral therapy	www.ccst.co.uk
Reflexology	www.reflexology.org
Sandra Cabot Liver Doctor	www.liverdoctor.com
Sandra Cabot Diet Doctor	www.weightcontroldoctor.com
Clay Body Wrap	www.universalcontourwrap.co.uk
Thyroid info	www.tpa-uk.org.uk

Appendix VII:
RECOMMENDED SUPPLIERS

Homeopathy	Helios Website: Helios.co.uk Telephone: 01892 546850 Ainsworth Pharmacy Website: Answorth.com Telephone: 020 7935 5330
Elixirs (US)	Website: Elixirs.com
Herbs	Neals Yard Website: Nealsyardremedies.com Telephone: 0845 2623145
Supplements	Metabolics Website: Metabolic.co.uk Telephone: 01380 812799 Nutri Website: Nutri.co.uk Telephone: 0800 212742 Nature's Sunshine (herbs as well as supplements) Website: Naturessunshine.co.uk Telephone: contact practitioners on website Solgar Website: solgar.co.uk

Ann Parker

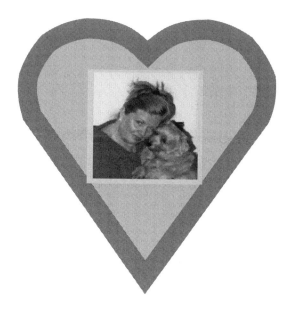

Ann Parker is a world renowned motivational speaker, weight loss expert, animal communicator and psychic behaviourist, psychic life coach, spiritual counsellor and healer. Ann has helped thousands of people lose weight and keep it off for life! Ann had a weight problem for nearly 60 years both being overweight and bulimic so she understands that these problems are very rarely anything to do with food. Ann knows that one treatment or one diet is not the answer so contained in this book is all the necessary components for you to lose weight FOREVER!

Ann works intuitively and psychically, she can work with a person anywhere in the world. Being psychic, Ann works on a much deeper level with spirit guides and angels and this is how she can modify patterns and blocks without even seeing the person.

This is a truly inspiring book, with amazing and funny stories, and successes interspersed between all the informative details. If you have a weight problem it is the only book you will ever need to read!

Printed in Great Britain
by Amazon

58511899R00229